AMERICAN JOURNAL of PUBLIC HEALTH
DECEMBER 2024
Issue 12

AJPH

A PUBLICATION OF THE
AMERICAN PUBLIC HEALTH ASSOCIATION

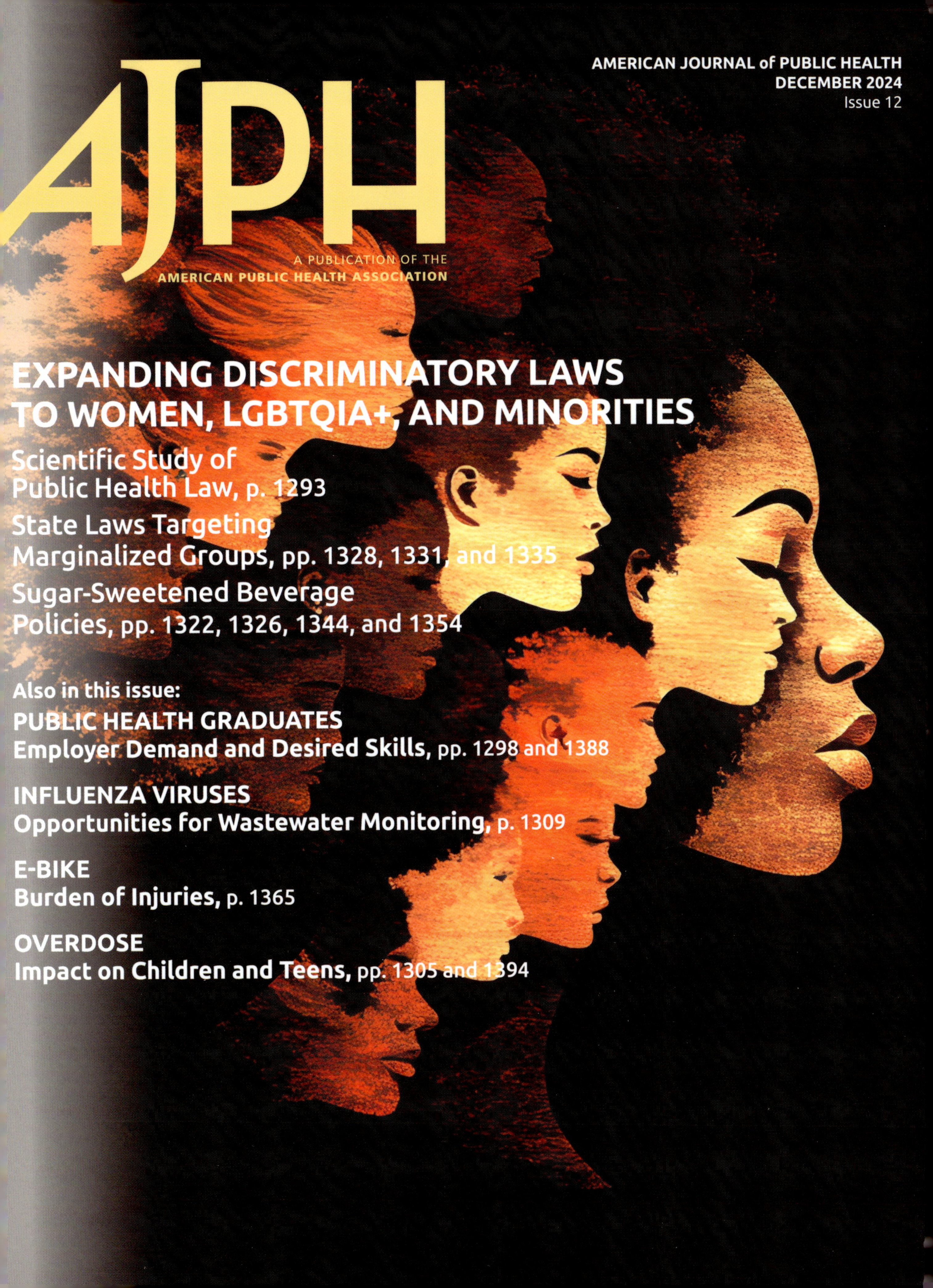

EXPANDING DISCRIMINATORY LAWS TO WOMEN, LGBTQIA+, AND MINORITIES

Scientific Study of Public Health Law, p. 1293

State Laws Targeting Marginalized Groups, pp. 1328, 1331, and 1335

Sugar-Sweetened Beverage Policies, pp. 1322, 1326, 1344, and 1354

Also in this issue:

PUBLIC HEALTH GRADUATES
Employer Demand and Desired Skills, pp. 1298 and 1388

INFLUENZA VIRUSES
Opportunities for Wastewater Monitoring, p. 1309

E-BIKE
Burden of Injuries, p. 1365

OVERDOSE
Impact on Children and Teens, pp. 1305 and 1394

AJPH®, published monthly, is the official Journal of the American Public Health Association®, 800 I St NW, Washington, DC 20001-3710; (202) 777- APHA; TDD (202) 777-2500. APHA is a nongovernmental professional society founded in 1872, representing all disciplines and specialties in public health.

The *American Journal of Public Health*® (*AJPH*) (print ISSN: 0090-0036; electronic ISSN: 1541- 0048), first published in 1911, is the official journal of the American Public Health Association® (APHA). The oldest and largest organization of public health professionals in the world, APHA represents approximately 30 000 members from more than 50 occupations of public health.

Submissions: Visit www.editorialmanager.com/ajph or ajph.edmgr.com for online manuscript preparation and submission guidelines. Contributions of original unpublished research, social science analyses, scholarly essays, critical commentaries, departments, and letters to the editor are welcome. Questions? Write ajph.submissions@apha.org or call APHA at (202) 777-2469.

Print plus online subscriptions: Institutional price (print copy with online access for a single institution and all authorized users, regardless of geographic location) varies by size of organization and ranges from $993–$1445 for US organizations, and $1073–$1526 for international organizations (air delivery); multiple campuses not permitted without special arrangement. Details of the tiered pricing system at https://subscriptionoffice.com/pages/apha-landing-page. To order, write apha.subscriptions@apha.org.

Online-only subscriptions: Institutional price for one institution and its authorized users (regardless of geographic location) is $878–$1307. To order, write apha.subscriptions@apha.org. For academic consortia or multisite corporate subscriptions, contact apha.subscriptions@apha.org.

Print-only subscriptions: Institutional price is US $701, $782 international.

Back print issues: A limited number of print issues are for sale. Single copies are US $49, $55 international (air delivery). Shipping included; prepay only. To order, write apha.subscriptions@apha.org.

Reprints: For prices and ordering information on 50 or more reprints, check the Reprints section at www.ajph.org. To order smaller quantities of reprints (rush delivery), use the "Purchase Article" link on the article site itself.

Electronic access: Online articles more than 10 years old are available free for personal use at www.ajph.org. Recent articles are available through pay-per-view: single PDF article for $24, single issue access for 24 hours for $33, or entire site access for 24 hours for $38.

Postal information: Periodicals postage paid at Washington, DC, and additional mailing offices. Postmaster: Send address changes to American Journal of Public Health, 800 I St NW, Washington, DC 20001-3710.

Address changes: Send to AJPH, Membership Department (members) or AJPH Subscriptions (subscribers), APHA, 800 I St NW, Washington, DC 20001-3710. Or write to membership.mail@apha. org (members) or apha.subscriptions@apha.org (subscribers).

Advertising: For pricing and other information, see www.ajph.org. Please write to ashell.alston@apha.org or call (202) 777-2470 for other advertising opportunities. Ask about special exhibit packages and sponsorships. Acceptance of advertising by the *Journal* does not imply endorsement of products.

Indexes: Publications that index or abstract articles from *AJPH* include the following: Ageline, Assia (Applied Social Science Index and Abstracts), Biological Abstracts, Chemical Abstracts, CINAHL, Criminal Justice Abstracts, EMBASE, EMCare, Environmental Abstracts, e-psyche, ERIC, ETOH (Alcohol and Alcohol Problems Science Database), Excerpta Medica, Food Science and Technology, General Science Index, Grateful Med, Hospital Literature Index, Human Resources Abstracts, International Pharmaceutical Abstracts (IPA), Medline, Physical Education Index, Pollution Abstracts, Psychological Abstracts, PsychINFO, Safety Science Abstracts, Sage Family Studies Abstracts, Sage Human Resources Abstracts, Science Citation Index, SCOPUS, SIIC Data Bases, Social Work Research and Abstracts, and Statistical Reference Index (SRI)/LexisNexis.

AJPH

A PUBLICATION OF THE
AMERICAN PUBLIC HEALTH ASSOCIATION

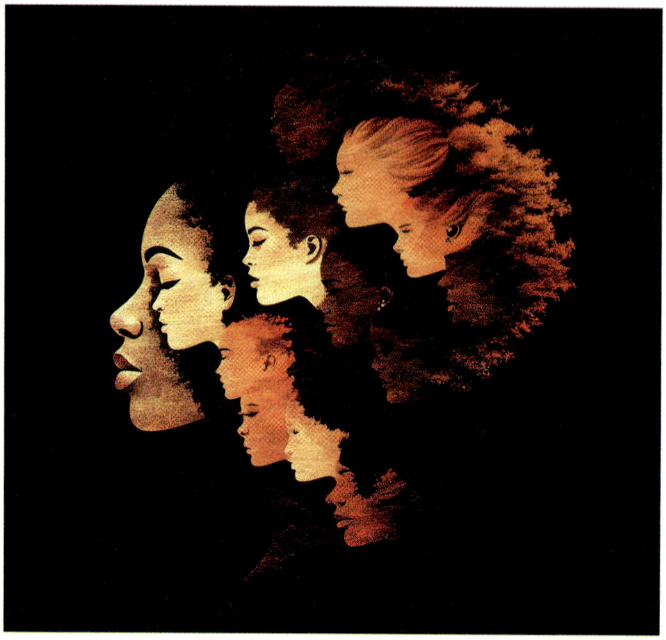

COVER: Socially marginalized groups are under attack. Discriminatory laws often viewed in isolation, focusing on a particular issue or group, actually overlap creating a synergistic health threat for vulnerable groups. The sweeping implications for public health can be traced back to more than 30 states that have enacted legislation since 2020 that targets Black people and other people of color, LGBTQIA+ people, transgender and nonbinary people, and women and other birthing people.

Cover concept and selection by Aleisha Kropf. Cover image by sunanta/ Adobe Stock. Printed with permission.

APHA
AMERICAN PUBLIC HEALTH ASSOCIATION
For science. For action. For health.

AJPH December 2024, Vol. 114, No. 12

Promoting public health research, policy, practice, and education is the *AJPH* mission. As we widen our scope to embrace global issues, we also sharpen our focus to support the needs of public health practitioners. We invite contributions of original unpublished research, opinion and commentary, and letters to the editor.

The *Journal* is printed on acid-free recycled paper.

OPEN ACCESS   ONLINE ONLY   PODCAST   DATA SUPPLEMENT AVAILABLE

EDITOR'S CHOICE

1293 The Promise of the Scientific Study of Public Health Law
W. E. Parmet

BOOKS & MEDIA

1295 Public Health Feminisms: Recognizing the Diversity of Experiences and Expertise
M. S. Parry

OPINIONS, IDEAS, & PRACTICE

EDITORIALS

1298 Bridging the Gap: Aligning Education for Public Health With Emerging Workforce Demands
L. Magaña and E. M. Burke

PERSPECTIVES

1300 Toward Community-Engaged Health Care to Bridge Public Health With Clinical Care
V. Guilamo-Ramos, F. K. Amankwah, R. Tucker-Seeley, V. B. B. Jernigan, and G. C. Benjamin

1305 The Call for a School-Based Approach to Opioid Overdose Prevention
J. B. Calihan, B. L. Carney, D. M. Schmill, and S. M. Bagley

1309 Challenges and Opportunities for Wastewater Monitoring of Influenza Viruses During the Multistate Outbreak of Highly Pathogenic Avian Influenza A(H5N1) Virus in Dairy Cattle and Poultry
M. A. Honein, S. J. Olsen, D. B. Jernigan, and D. C. Daskalakis

1313 Tracking Airborne Lead Exposures That Disrupt Children's Fronto-executive Functions and Inhibitory Systems
L. S. Neuwirth

NOTES FROM THE FIELD

1317 Breaking Down Silos Within a Multihospital System: Lessons From the California Department of State Hospitals' Response to the COVID-19 Pandemic
M. I. Ventura, R. Schaufenbil, T. Do, J. C. Arguello, J. Siegel, and K. Warburton

STATE LAWS TARGETING MARGINALIZED GROUPS

1322 Media Communications Must Promote Healthy Hydration Policies and Environments That Encourage Water Consumption to Reduce Sugary Beverage Health Risks
V. I. Kraak and N. L. Furr

1326 A Treasure Trove Inventory of Sugar-Sweetened Beverage Policies in the United States, 2014–2023
E. Crosbie and L. Schmidt

1328 All Hands on Deck: Addressing Obstacles to Applying an Intersectionality Framework in Health Research
D. M. Crookes

1331 The Return of Jim Crow: Government Discrimination Against Women, LGBTQIA+ Individuals, and Racial/Ethnic Minority Individuals
R. Yearby

RESEARCH & ANALYSIS

STATE LAWS TARGETING MARGINALIZED GROUPS

1335 The Synergistic Health Threats of State Laws Targeting Marginalized Groups in the United States
K. Underhill, V. A. Earnshaw, and K. M. Nelson

1344 An Inventory of Proposed and Enacted Sugar-Sweetened Beverage Policies at the State, Local, and Tribal Levels in the United States, 2014–2023
J. N. Davis, S. Goon, J. Gouck, S. E. Solar, S. Mancini, A. M. Ortega Hinojosa, J. Krieger, and J. Falbe

1354 Countermarketing Versus Health Education Messages About Sugar-Sweetened Beverages: An Online Randomized Controlled Trial of US Adults
A. H. Grummon, A. B. Zeitlin, C. J. Y. Lee, M. G. Hall, C. Collis, L. P. Cleveland, and J. Petimar

HEALTH MONITORING

1365 The Burden of Injuries Associated With E-Bikes, Powered Scooters, Hoverboards, and Bicycles in the United States: 2019–2022
K. G. Burford, N. G. Itzkowitz, A. G. Rundle, C. DiMaggio, and S. J. Mooney

1375 Assessment of Health Disparities and Sexual Orientation Response Choices Used in Two US National Population-Based Health Surveys, 2020–2021
N. F. Kahn, C. T. Halpern, D. R. Burshell, S. M. Hernandez, and K. J. Conron

1384 Levels and Changes in Defensive Firearm Use by US Crime Victims, 1987–2021
D. McDowall, B. Wiersema, C. Loftin, and R. McCleary

OPEN-THEMED RESEARCH

1388 Employer Demand and Desired Skills for Public Health Graduates: Evidence From Job Postings
H. Krasna

1394 More Than 1.4 Million US Children Have Lost a Family Member to Drug Overdose
A. M. Verdery, C. Ryan-Claytor, E. Smith-Greenaway, N. Sarkar, and M. Livings

1398 Food Industry Compliance With the Display of Front-of-Package Warning Labels at the Final Phase (2020) of Chile's Labeling and Advertising Law
N. Rebolledo, P. Ferrer-Rosende, M. Reyes, L. S. Taillie, and C. Corvalán

BACKMATTER

OTHER DEPARTMENTS

1408 Subscription Form

1st

We were the first school of public health in the U.S.

10%

Ranked in the top 10% of schools and programs of public health in the U.S.

INSIGHT Into Diversity
HIGHER EDUCATION EXCELLENCE IN DIVERSITY AWARD
2023
Health Professions School

Thanks to her continuing support, our school is proud to be renamed:

TULANE UNIVERSITY
Celia Scott Weatherhead School *of* Public Health & Tropical Medicine

Established in 1912 and rebranded in 2024, the Celia Scott Weatherhead School of Public Health continues to educate passionate students who want to make a difference in the health and well-being of populations around the globe. Located in New Orleans our school is at the epicenter of some of the most pressing issues facing public health today, like the intersection of climate change and health, the intractability of health inequities, and the re-emergence of tropical infectious diseases.

We are **the** public health school of the South and a leader globally.

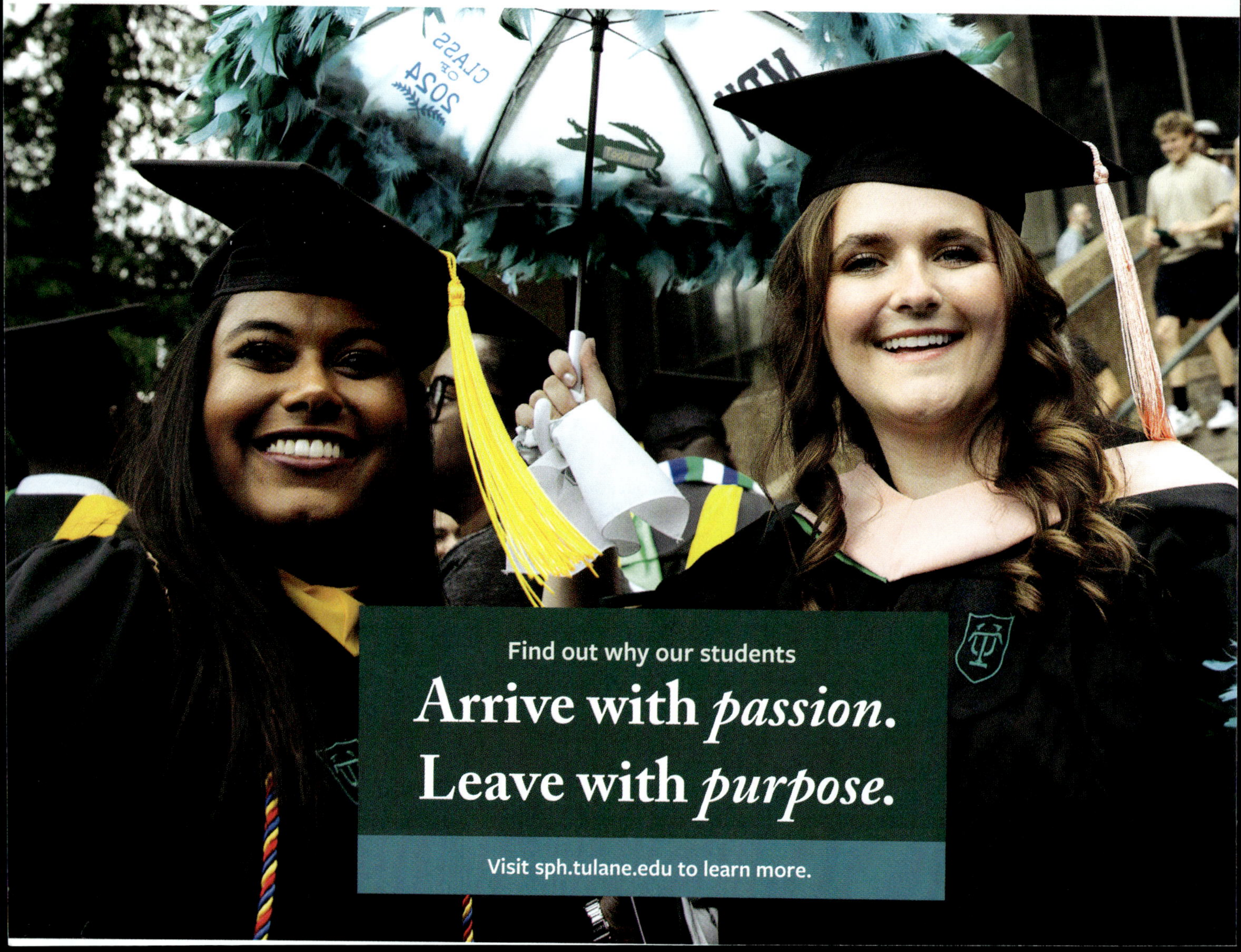

The Promise of the Scientific Study of Public Health Law

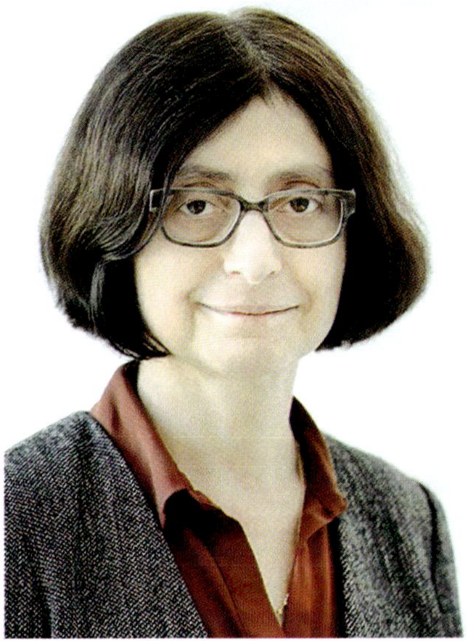

Wendy E. Parmet, JD
Associate Editor, *AJPH*

Despite law's importance to public health, until relatively recently, researchers seldom studied law's impact on health with the same scientific rigor they apply to other phenomena that affect health.

Laws are the means through which many public health policies are effectuated or undermined. Statutes, ordinances, and regulations, issued by governments at all levels, can codify or preclude health policies, such as those established by the Affordable Care Act. Laws also grant or limit health officials' authority to develop, implement, and enforce health measures, such as quarantine orders. Judicial decisions also have a significant effect on health, as was apparent by the Supreme Court's overruling of *Roe v Wade*.

Previously, health policy researchers frequently studied the consequences of policies without focusing on the legal context in which those policies were implemented. Conversely, most public health law scholars analyzed and contextualized legal texts without using the tools of science to study the impact or prevalence of a particular law.

Fortunately, as the articles published by *AJPH* over the past several years demonstrate, and as the articles in the current special section showcase, the study of law's relationship to public health has become more sophisticated. In part, this is attributable to advances in legal epidemiology. The Centers for Disease Control and Prevention defines this as "the study of law as a factor in the cause, distribution, and prevention of disease and injury" and notes that it "applies rigorous, scientific methods to translate complex legal language into data that can be used to evaluate how laws affect population health" (https://bit.ly/4gRIrhd). Legal epidemiology can also be used to compile and map positive laws, such as statutes, regulations, and administrative opinions, as evident in the two lead articles in this special section (Davis et al., p. 1344, examining sugary beverage laws; Underhill et al., p. 1335, examining laws targeting marginalized populations).

Although neither article empirically studies the health effects of the laws they discuss, their findings shine a light

Continued on page 1294...

HISTORY CORNER

57 YEARS AGO

[A] new pattern in federal health legislation has emerged. A systematic and integrated approach rather than a piece-meal approach can be adopted now to ensure optimal contribution to the nation's health by the federal government. The system will include support of the total range of health services and resources: basic education, specialty training, research and service facilities, continuing education, preventive and curative programs, and service monies for vendor payment. Now, by involvement in the entire array of factors pertinent to the health of the nation, the federal government can approach health problems comprehensively, and thereby fulfill its public mandates more fully and effectively than in the past.

From *AJPH*, June 1967, p. 941

on important trends and developments. For example, Underhill et al. show that a majority of states that have enacted laws targeting one marginalized group in the past few years have enacted laws targeting other groups as well. Likewise, the database of Davis et al. shows that the enactment of laws aimed at reducing the consumption of sugary beverages has slowed in recent years. As Crosbie and Schmidt (p. 1326) and Crookes (p. 1328) note, such studies can help researchers study the public health implications of state statutes.

The articles published in the special section also illustrate another positive development in the study of law's relationship to public health: the increased focus on equity and the incorporation of social science theories, including critical race and intersectionality theories. For example, Yearby (p. 1331) uses a critical race lens to assess the impact of state laws targeting marginalized groups, and Underhill et al. present a logic model that can be used to examine how laws can interact with other social determinants of health to shape inequities. And in her article, Crookes offers recommendations that epidemiologists and social scientists can use to study the interactive impact of multiple systems of oppression.

Such articles exemplify the increasing sophistication and promise of the scientific study of public health law. Ideally, as Crosbie and Schmidt suggest in their article, this can lead to the development of policies and laws that offer stronger protection for health and equity. Less optimistically, the articles in the current section and others published by *AJPH* over the past several years also show that the trends are not all positive. A richer and more rigorous understanding of law's influence on health, it seems, is not sufficient to ensure better health. We also need to understand how to influence the political, economic, and cultural forces that seek to block law's capacity to improve health and redress inequities. AJPH

DOI: https://doi.org/10.2105/AJPH.2024.307885

ORCID iD:
Wendy E. Parmet https://orcid.org/0000-0002-5797-0863

HISTORY CORNER

106 YEARS AGO

Maine's New Health Law

At the adjournment of the seventy-eighth legislature of the state of Maine on April 7 the newspapers commented at length upon its acts relating to war, suffrage and prohibition, but nothing was said about a matter no less important to a modern democracy: namely, public health. . . . The act creating a State Department of Health was introduced and supported by the State Medical Association. . . . The task of the new department is not an easy one but it is confidently hoped that this type of organization which has been instituted in New York and Massachusetts with highly satisfactory results, being continued from year to year with its original freedom from political system and with a general cooperation for increased efficiency, may yield to Maine all that it has given to these other States in decreasing the amount of preventable disease and promoting the health of its citizens.

From *AJPH*, May 1917, pp. 502, 504

Public Health Feminisms: Recognizing the Diversity of Experiences and Expertise

Manon S. Parry, PhD

ABOUT THE AUTHOR

Manon S. Parry is with the Department of History, European Studies, and Religious Studies at the University of Amsterdam, the Netherlands.

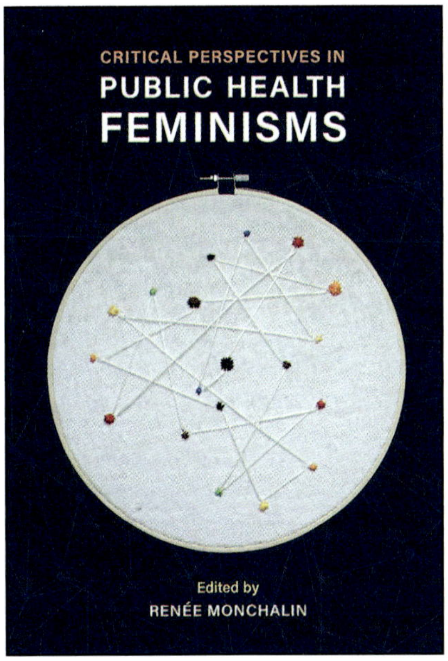

Critical Perspectives in Public Health Feminisms
By Renée Monachlin, ed.
Ontario, Canada: Canadian Scholars; 2023
292 pp.; CA $62.95
ISBN: 978-1773383569

As a research assistant for an Indigenous-led action research center, editor Renée Monachlin learned that "communities outside of the mainstream held effective and locally tailored public health knowledges and methods that worked" (p. 3), although she had never encountered such examples in her university education—which instead focused on canonical examples and (mythologized) figures.[1] This book, and the associated course Public Health Feminisms at the University of Victoria, aims to support "students and researchers alike to reveal and unpack how public health in Canada is a direct reflection of the country's very own beginnings—that of patriarchy and colonialism" (p. 3). The collection will also be of interest beyond Canada, especially in settler–colonial contexts, and consists of 16 chapters by a total of 52 authors, including many women of color, with an introduction and conclusion by the editor and contributions from students from undergraduate through the doctoral level, as well as academic researchers with public health roles. The essays provide compelling examples of public health feminist research and practice on mental health (Chapter 4); reproductive health (Chapters 5, 7, and 9); housing (Chapter 15); ableism, sexism, and racism in education (Chapters 6, 13, 14); and diversifying the profession (Chapters 2, 3, and 11).[2]

Cover artwork was created by Matsko Friedland, "a young urban Métis woman coming from a working-class family" (p. 2), and was produced as her final assignment for the Public Health Feminisms course. Her introductory remarks explaining its significance set the tone for the essays that follow. The white piece of towel used as the basis for the embroidery represents "the existing foundation of public health on which we build public health futures: predominantly white, timeworn, and in desperate need of replacement or repair" (p. xiii). The colors of the sewn dots come from the Philadelphia Pride flag, the first to incorporate black and brown stripes, representing "queer black and brown people . . . to recognize some of the groups who continue to be disproportionally affected by negative health outcomes" (p. xiii).

DIVERSIFYING SYLLABI

The chapters "bring together voices from Canadian public health disciplines that are often silenced: Black, Indigenous, racialized, refugee, immigrant, neurodiverse, disabled, two-spirit, nonbinary, trans and/or gender-diverse, and/or other marginalized/oppressed women" (p. 5). Themes include "intersectionality, knowledge sharing, reciprocity, the social determinants of health" (p. xiii), and the collection provides a useful primer on positionality, gender equality and equity, and racism, and introduces students to approaches including Black feminism, reproductive justice, and a "feminist ethic of care" (p. 165).

The style is consistent with a core course text, and all chapters begin with a list of learning objectives and end with "critical thinking questions," key terms, and suggested further readings. Theoretical concepts and intersectional approaches are explained in side-bar text boxes, including activism, social movements, and public health and gender and (dis)ability, as well as some highlighted events in the history of public health. Although terms such as ableism are well explained, other evolving or contested language, such as cisgender[3] and neurotypical,[4] are defined and used without attention to such flux, meaning that critical reflection on terms and their consequences is uneven.

LESSONS OF HISTORY

The authors integrate a variety of elements that highlight the purpose and value of challenging disciplinary conventions, including poetry and storytelling. Historical perspectives are also drawn upon to contextualize current issues as legacies, continuities, or consequences of the past. While this can be highly illuminating, the compression of complex histories into such short summaries also obscures important aspects and simplifies developments, sometimes unhelpfully. The extremely foreshortened history of feminism in the editor's introductory essay is one example, where each wave is summed up in an abbreviated characterization, written from a presentist perspective, contradicting a key point noted elsewhere in the collection, that "there has never been a universally agreed agenda for feminism" (p. 18) nor, in fact, a comprehensive history of the variety of groups and activities involved.[5]

The significance of historical events for contemporary health issues is nevertheless made powerfully salient in many of the chapters, including "Spurring the Witch Hunt: Abortion, Colonialism, Stigma, and Indigenous Knowledges in Canada," which examines contemporary stigma surrounding abortion as a product of the historical legacies of the suppression of Indigenous knowledge about birth limitation and the more recent and ongoing undermining of reproductive self-determination through forced sterilization and coerced abortion (p. 57–67). This essay does a particularly good job of demonstrating how harm can be perpetuated even by those attempting to help or heal others.

The historical overview in the opening pages of Chapter 10, "Strangers in our Homeland: The Impact of Racism Across Healthcare Policy and Delivery for Indigenous Peoples in Canada," is less effective, although the rest of the essay powerfully demonstrates how hidden histories play out today in devastating ways (p. 133–143). Although the discussion of the terrible array of abuses perpetuated by colonial settlers notes that seeing others as lesser or less-than humans led to genocidal and inhumane acts, the role of well-intentioned health professionals in this work is obfuscated by a focus on "governmental systems . . . trying to harm Indigenous Peoples" (p. 134). Chapter 12, "Reclamation of Matriarchy and Kinship Systems," usefully examines this aspect in more detail, focusing on the removal of Indigenous children from their families in the residential school system of the 19th and early 20th century, as well as the practice of placing children with non-Indigenous parents from the 1950s to the 1980s, and the foster care system today (p. 155–163).

CHALLENGING REDUCTIONISM

Several essays offer examples of applying public health feminist methods in research design, notably "Stuck in a High Wire Act: Ways of Understanding Immigrant Women's Mental Health Beyond Biomedicine" (p. 39–56). Postcolonial narrative inquiry is presented as a method to "counter damaging master narratives, decenter colonialist epistemologies, and challenge epistemic violence" with interview results presented and analyzed to demonstrate the range of factors that create "migratory distress," and that are obscured by reductionist diagnoses of depression and anxiety (p. 42). "Black Feminism in Critical Public Health Research, Policy, and Programming: Theory and Practice for Promoting the Health and Well-Being of Black Women" is another example, which additionally includes policy consideration and recommendations (p. 99–117).

Overall, the collection does a good job of demonstrating the value of reflecting upon the impact of individual experience, educational priorities, and structural inequalities on one's own work, and of reforming the public health system, from education and career trajectories to research and practice. There is some repetition if read as a whole, and some readers may find the weaknesses highlighted here counterproductive to the goal of advancing critical perspectives, but these issues could be easily addressed by assigning this text alongside a diverse array of readings and case studies, which is precisely what the editor hoped for. AJPH

CORRESPONDENCE

Correspondence should be sent to Manon S. Parry, Department of History, European Studies, and Religious Studies, University of Amsterdam, PO Box 1610, 1000 BP Amsterdam, The Netherlands (e-mail: m.s.parry@uva.nl). Reprints can be ordered at https://www.ajph.org by clicking the "Reprints" link.

PUBLICATION INFORMATION

Full Citation: Parry MS. Public Health Feminisms: recognizing the diversity of experiences and expertise. *Am J Public Health*. 2024;114(12): 1295–1297.

Acceptance Date: July 7, 2024.

DOI: https://doi.org/10.2105/AJPH.2024.307835

ORCID iD:

Manon S. Parry https://orcid.org/0000-0001-8369-2708

CONFLICTS OF INTEREST

The author reports no conflicts of interest.

REFERENCES

1. Koch T. John Snow, hero of cholera: RIP. *CMAJ*. 2008;178(13):1736. https://doi.org/10.1503/cmaj.080805
2. Hammarström A. Why feminism in public health? *Scand J Public Health*. 1999;27(4):241–244. https://doi.org/10.1177/14034948990270040601
3. Esacove A. Common patterns of cisgender use in public health articles and their implications for gender inclusivity efforts, 2013–2020. *Am J Public Health*. 2024;114(2):202–208. https://doi.org/10.2105/AJPH.2023.307441
4. Runswick-Cole K. (2014). 'Us' and 'them': the limits and possibilities of a 'politics of neurodiversity' in neoliberal times. *Disabil Soc*. 2020;29(7):1117–1129. https://doi.org/10.1080/09687599.2014.910107
5. Gamble S, ed. *The Routledge Critical Dictionary of Feminism and Postfeminism*. New York NY: Routledge; 2000: viii.

Bridging the Gap: Aligning Education for Public Health With Emerging Workforce Demands

Laura Magaña, MSc, PhD, and Emily M. Burke, EdD, MPH

ABOUT THE AUTHORS

Laura Magaña is the president and chief executive officer of the Association of Schools and Programs of Public Health (ASPPH), Washington, DC. Emily M. Burke is the senior director, ASPPH Center for Public Health Workforce Development.

See also Krasna, p. 1388.

AJPH December 2024, Vol. 114, No. 12

With global health challenges and technological advancements rapidly reshaping public health, the urgency and necessity of aligning educational programs with real-world expectations are paramount. The increasing demand for public health professionals necessitates academic training that equips future leaders with the practical skills to address evolving challenges and employer demands. The dynamic job market presents a crucial opportunity for education in public health to innovate and transform, with curricula strategically aligned to current workforce trends and demands.

THE INTERSECTION OF ACADEMIA AND THE JOB MARKET

Public health degree programs are pivotal in preparing practitioners to promote health, prevent disease, and engage with diverse communities to advance health equity. As essential public health services evolve, there is an increasing focus on leadership and systems thinking, effective communication, community engagement and partnership, policy and advocacy, data science, and health equity (https://bit.ly/3YoTdEJ). These training areas highlight the importance of equipping public health graduates with both traditional expertise and modern competencies in equal measure.

Given the emergence of new competencies and necessary skills, fueled in part by the COVID-19 pandemic, education for public health must align curricula with current workforce trends and employer demands.[1] Educational and theoretical frameworks that adapt to changes in public health practice are crucial for preparing graduates for interprofessional opportunities across various industries and job sectors.[2,3] Furthermore, as evidenced by an analysis of job postings for MPH graduates by Krasna in this issue of *AJPH* (p. 1388), the Council on Education for Public Health has a unique opportunity in the upcoming 2026 criteria revision to establish competencies that address both core and specialized technical job requirements.

IDENTIFYING AND ADDRESSING COMPETENCY GAPS

Identifying and addressing competency gaps in education for public health will require exploring existing education and labor data and intentional collaboration between academia and practice to assess current public health curriculum and degree delivery alongside required job skills and responsibilities. Association of Schools and Programs of Public Health (ASPPH) proposes a systematic process to identify training gaps using available resources, including the recent ASPPH Governmental Public Health Job Task Analysis, the de Beaumont Foundation's Public Health Workforce Interests and Needs Survey, the Public Health Foundation's Core Competencies for Public Health Professionals, and the Council on Education for Public Health's Foundational Competencies for Public Health Bachelor's, MPH, and DrPH degrees. Furthermore, while ASPPH has a robust data set on the first-destination outcomes of graduates of schools and programs of public health,[4] our field lacks systematic data collection to observe the career trajectories and identify the continuing education needs of public health practitioners. ASPPH has proposed such a system and is in the process of developing an implementation strategy.

Ultimately, however, academic public health must engage with public health employers and develop strategies to operationalize what is learned through applied practice experiences and in the classroom. Emphasizing case-based and active learning in tandem with ongoing collaboration with practitioners and employers to update competencies and incorporate technological advancements (e.g., machine learning and artificial intelligence), will help develop a more adaptable and skilled workforce.[5]

Executed within the frameworks of Public Health 3.0 and the 10 Essential Public Health Services, as well as the ASPPH Framing the Future 2030 initiative, this approach will address complex social determinants of health and multisector engagement to generate collective impact. Furthermore, centering inclusivity, equity, adaptability, and continuous innovation ensures that graduates are equipped to lead in a rapidly changing global environment.[6]

To bridge the gap between public health competencies and job demands, education for public health will need to emphasize and balance value-driven approaches with technological advancements. This includes fostering interdisciplinary research, such as collaborations between public health professionals and data scientists for predictive disease models, and enhancing community engagement through diverse initiatives like community health worker programs focused on community health promotion.[7]

ENHANCING EDUCATION FOR PUBLIC HEALTH

Enhancing education for public health with insights from employers goes beyond closing gaps; it involves the refinement of core competencies and the development of specialized competencies to prepare graduates to embrace technology for leadership and innovation. Global and local perspectives provide innovative practices for curriculum updates, while education for public health offers models for incorporating cutting-edge technologies and addressing emerging health challenges.[2] Cultivating and fostering partnerships with public health practitioners and employers can enhance educational relevance and effectiveness, equipping graduates to lead and innovate in a complex field.[8] In addition, integrating education and labor data; focusing on technical skills, microcredentials, and certifications; and adapting curricula to reflect emerging trends can significantly boost graduates' employability and effectiveness.[2]

To stay ahead in a rapidly evolving field, education for public health must embrace both technological advancements and real-world demands. By aligning curricula with job market trends and integrating essential core and emerging competencies, academic public health can better prepare graduates to thrive in an ever-changing world. This proactive alignment ensures that education for public health remains relevant, responsive, and effective in addressing both present and future challenges. AJPH

CORRESPONDENCE

Correspondence should be sent to Laura Magaña, 1900 M Street NW, Suite 710, Washington, DC 20036 (e-mail: lmagana@aspph.org). Reprints can be ordered at https://ajph.org by clicking the "Reprints" link.

PUBLICATION INFORMATION

Full Citation: Magaña L, Burke EM. Bridging the gap: aligning education for public health with emerging workforce demands. *Am J Public Health*. 2024;114(12):1298–1299.

Acceptance Date: September 18, 2024.

DOI: https://doi.org/10.2105/AJPH.2024.307871

ORCID iDs:

Laura Magaña https://orcid.org/0000-0002-6767-4339

Emily M. Burke https://orcid.org/0000-0001-5534-5100

CONTRIBUTORS

L. Magaña served as the lead author for this editorial, drafting the initial version, which laid the foundation for the key arguments and perspectives presented. Her work included conceptualizing the structure and framing the overall narrative, ensuring the editorial aligned with the intended focus of the publication. E. M. Burke contributed significantly to the editorial by thoroughly revising the draft, expanding upon the original ideas, and incorporating additional references to strengthen the arguments. Her revisions added clarity, depth, and broader context, ensuring the editorial was comprehensive and well-supported by relevant literature. Both authors were involved in the final review and approved the article for submission.

ACKNOWLEDGMENTS

Special thanks to the editorial team of *AJPH* for their thoughtful feedback and guidance throughout the revision process.

CONFLICTS OF INTEREST

The authors declare no potential or actual conflicts of interest related to the funding, affiliations, or activities associated with this editorial. Both authors are employed by ASPPH, but this affiliation did not influence the content or direction of the editorial.

REFERENCES

1. Sullivan LM, Weist EM, Barrington WE, et al. Education for public health 2030: transformation to meet health needs in a changing world. *Front Public Health*. 2023;11:1269272. https://doi.org/10.3389/fpubh.2023.1269272
2. Frenk J, Chen LC, Chandran L, et al. Challenges and opportunities for educating health professionals after the COVID-19 pandemic. *Lancet*. 2022;400(10362):1539–1556. https://doi.org/10.1016/S0140-6736(22)02092-X
3. Salmon JW. Profit and health care: trends in corporatization and proprietarization. In: *The Corporate Transformation of Health Care*. Oxfordshire, England: Routledge; 2020:55–77.
4. Plepys CM, Krasna H, Leider JP, Burke EM, Blakely CH, Magaña L. First-destination outcomes for 2015–2018 public health graduates: focus on employment. *Am J Public Health*. 2021;111(3):475–484. https://doi.org/10.2105/AJPH.2020.306038
5. Yudell M, Amon JJ. What's next for public health? Health Affairs Forefront; 2024. Available at: https://www.healthaffairs.org/content/forefront/s-next-public-health. Accessed October 9, 2024.
6. *The Transformative Approaches to Teaching and Learning Report. Framing the Future 2030: Education for Public Health*. Washington, DC: Association of Schools and Programs of Public Health; March 2024.
7. Krasna H, Kornfeld J, Cushman L, Ni S, Antoniou P, March D. The new public health workforce: employment outcomes of public health graduate students. *J Public Health Manag Pract*. 2021;27(1):12–19. https://doi.org/10.1097/PHH.0000000000000976
8. Lee S, Yoon JY, Hwang Y. Collaborative project-based learning in global health: enhancing competencies and skills for undergraduate nursing students. *BMC Nurs*. 2024;23(1):437. https://doi.org/10.1186/s12912-024-02111-8

Toward Community-Engaged Health Care to Bridge Public Health With Clinical Care

Vincent Guilamo-Ramos, PhD, MPH, LCSW, ANP-BC, PMHNP-BC, Francis K. Amankwah, MPH, Reginald Tucker-Seeley, ScD, ScM, MA, Valarie Blue Bird Jernigan, DrPH, MPH, and Georges C. Benjamin, MD

ABOUT THE AUTHORS

Vincent Guilamo-Ramos is with the Institute for Policy Solutions, Johns Hopkins University School of Nursing, Washington, DC. Francis K. Amankwah is with the National Academies of Sciences, Engineering, and Medicine, Washington, DC. Reginald Tucker-Seely is with Health Equity Strategies and Solutions, Los Angeles, CA. Valarie Blue Bird Jernigan is with the Center for Indigenous Health Research and Policy, Oklahoma State University Center for Health Sciences, Tulsa. Georges C. Benjamin is with the American Public Health Association, Washington, DC. All of the authors served on the Adhoc National Academies of Sciences, Engineering, and Medicine Committee on Unequal Treatment Revisited: The Current State of Racial and Ethnic Disparities in Healthcare.

AJPH December 2024, Vol. 114, No. 12

Approximately 20 years ago, the Institute of Medicine, now the National Academy of Medicine, released *Unequal Treatment: Confronting Racial and Ethnic Disparities in Health Care* (commonly known as the *Unequal Treatment* report).[1] That report concluded that pervasive health inequities (referred to as health disparities) have been burdening racially and ethnically minoritized populations within the United States.[1] The report revealed that a key driver of these inequities was structural and systemic racism and provided recommendations to eliminate health care inequities. That landmark report—arguably one of the most important health policy reports ever undertaken—provided a roadmap and call to action for our nation to make progress in addressing historical health inequities that were deeply embedded in the process of health care and reflected in the fabric of broader US society.[1]

In June 2024, the National Academies of Sciences, Engineering, and Medicine released a 20-year follow-up to the original *Unequal Treatment* report. This most recent report, *Ending Unequal Treatment: Strategies to Achieve Equitable Health Care and Optimal Health for All,* evaluates the current state of health care in the United States regarding racially and ethnically minoritized populations.[2] In addition, the report committee explored what progress, if any, the United States has made in the elimination of health inequities since 2003.[2] If progress has been achieved, what are some of the reasons behind this progress? If the United States has made inadequate progress, what can explain the lack of progress? Most importantly, the *Ending Unequal Treatment* report[2] identifies the existing evidence for advancing the nation's quest to eliminate health care inequities and bolster both health care and broader societal health equity.[2]

The *Ending Unequal Treatment* report provided several recommendations for public health and health care delivery systems. In this *AJPH* editorial, we seek to address one key overarching conclusion of the report: the US health care system overly relies on the most costly diagnostic and treatment procedures focused on the management of disease, with inadequate attention given to how the health care system can be leveraged to better advance wellness, prevention, and health promotion in ways that are equitable and optimal for all. This dominant approach results in a health care system that suboptimally addresses the health and health-related social needs of our nation.

The disruption of the health care system is most evident among racially and ethnically minoritized communities. However, the spillover effects of our current approach have implications for the entire population. We underscore the urgency of advancing new models of primary care to strengthen population health and eliminate health inequities. The implementation of this recommendation will require individual, organizational, and systemic changes to the health care delivery system.

PREVENTION AND HEALTH PROMOTION VS DISEASE TREATMENT

The United States currently has a health care system that is overly focused on the provision of sick care, which can be defined as health care that prioritizes the management and treatment of disease versus prioritization of wellness, prevention, and health promotion.[2] The United States expends far more financial resources on the provision of health care than other countries in the world.[3] However, we consistently report worse health and health care outcomes than other developed nations and, increasingly, certain developing nations.[2,3]

The United States spends approximately $4.8 trillion on health care for costs primarily allocated to treating disease.[3,4] The sole type of health care that has the potential for improving population health—primary care—is the segment of health care that receives the least amount of investment,[2] despite its crucial role in supporting our nation's health.[5] The primary care system is underresourced and often overburdened with diagnosing, treating, and managing disease, with much less attention given to supporting wellness, preventing illness, and promoting health.[6] The inability of the primary care system to better address population health and wellness has resulted in an increasingly costly health care system[3,4] that overly utilizes the costliest procedures[6] and misses its greatest potential: elevating the health of our entire nation.

A health status snapshot of the overall US population highlights troublesome trends; for example, most adults 18 years and older in the United States have one or more largely preventable chronic conditions, and 63% of people 65 years and older live with multiple chronic conditions.[7] In addition, over the past decade, life expectancy has on average decreased or stagnated[8] relative to the extent of the financial expenditures associated with our costly health care system and relative to other nations where greater investments in social care have been well integrated into traditional clinical care.[3,4] As a notable exemplar, the Indian Health Service, which is responsible for providing federal health services to the American Indian and Alaska Native population, is chronically underfunded and meets less than half of the health care needs of the population.[9] This contributes to the lower life expectancy of American Indians and Alaska Natives, approximately eight years less than that of the general US population.[8]

Furthermore, projections regarding the future population health status of our nation highlight a trajectory characterized by increasing numbers of individuals developing one or more chronic diseases.[2,7] The effects of chronic disease on the overall well-being and financial stability of the United States cannot be understated.[10] The current trajectory is unsustainable and has far-reaching implications for US households as well as the overall health of the population and the economic stability of our nation.[11] Of dire concern are the billions of dollars that health economists identify as the costs we contribute to maintaining an inequitable health care system.[12] The country desperately needs a paradigm shift: a reimagined model of care that more fully integrates clinical care centered on prevention and health promotion while also embedding social care into an integrated model of health service provision that bridges public health and primary care.

According to the *Ending Unequal Treatment* report, greater investments in Centers for Medicare & Medicaid Services Section 1115 Health Related Social Needs Demonstration projects are promising and should be further scaled up.[2,13] These projects use Medicaid dollars to address the health-related social needs of program participants. Preliminary evidence suggests that there are promising outcomes regarding cost savings, reductions in unnecessary emergency room visits and hospitalizations, and strengthening of community-based organizations now receiving Medicaid dollars for service provision.[2,13,14] Receipt of these Medicaid reimbursement funds has provided transformative revenue and infrastructure to community-based organizations traditionally not eligible for these funds.[2,14] In addition, the workforce employed by these organizations has been more readily conceptualized as essential for interprofessional health care team members.

COMMUNITY-ENGAGED CLINICAL AND SOCIAL CARE

Health inequities reflect unjust and unfair negative health outcomes that are most noticeably observed in minoritized and marginalized populations.[2] Furthermore, health care inequities reveal the deliberate and unconscious ways in which health care systems and providers allocate services and deliver care.[2] Health care inequities occur within a broader context of health inequity and are inextricably tied to the social environments where people live, learn, work, and play (i.e. the social and structural determinants of health), and they involve both the tangible provision of public goods and services such as housing and education and social processes such as systemic and structural racism and anti-immigrant sentiment that are embedded throughout health care systems and broader society.[15–17]

The distinction between health care inequities and health inequities is meaningful and warrants consideration regarding how a novel, more effective primary care system could be designed to better integrate both clinical and social care into a robust delivery system across multiple levels, including the individual provider–patient level and the health care institutional level. Also, there is a need to adopt broader societal policies related to health and social welfare.[2]

Eliminating health care inequities will necessitate a sustained commitment to this effort, readiness to implement systemic change within health care, and meaningful engagement of the communities that health care systems are intended to serve. This mandate is most evident in the lack of meaningful engagement of racially and ethnically minoritized groups who experience the majority of the health care inequities observed in the current US health care system.[2] Meaningful engagement moves well beyond cursory community advisory groups and other more performative mechanisms for eliciting superficial input from racially and ethnically minoritized groups.[2,18,19] Rather, meaningful engagement requires a commitment to the deliberate alignment of the health care system to the needs of the communities served.[2,18,19] This alignment is built on a set of principles and practices that reflect equal levels of power, trustworthiness, willingness to allocate financial incentives to all partners in equitable ways, and willingness to address how, where, by whom, and what kind of health care is provided.[18–20]

Given the horrific racial/ethnic morbidity and mortality inequities our nation endured, the COVID-19 pandemic again reminded us of the importance of meaningful community engagement for public health. However, is the health care delivery system ready for the systemic change required to adequately engage with communities and sustain health care inequity interventions? Lack of individual and organizational readiness for change within the health care delivery system may hamper such efforts.

Nevertheless, numerous articles published in *AJPH*[18,19,21] have highlighted the instrumental role of community engagement in eliminating health inequities and the profession's endorsement of a paradigm shift away from a health system with unilateral delivery of health services to a deliberate and committed partnership between health systems, communities, nonprofit organizations, and other stakeholders. At the heart of a newly envisioned partnership with communities are trusted relationships[17–21] in which communities perceive that their best interests are reflected in the actions, programs, and policies implemented within their local health systems. The *Ending Unequal Treatment* report highlights the need for our health care system to move away from episodic and sporadic care to a predictable "relationship-based" system characterized by person-centered and whole-person care.[2]

REDEFINING THE HEALTH CARE WORKFORCE

Currently, the US health care workforce is too narrowly defined. Historically, the health care workforce has been conceptualized as consisting of primarily clinicians such as physicians, nurses, and pharmacists.[2] Too often, interprofessional health care workforce team members' contributions to eliminating health inequities are omitted.[22] For example, there is compelling evidence that community health workers, social workers, behavioral health and addiction providers, and so forth are highly effective members of the health care workforce.[22] Despite compelling data on the important contributions of these health care workforce team members, dominant models of health care delivery underprioritize their utilization in eliminating health inequities.[2,22] This is most notable in the lack of reimbursement for services provided by community health workers and other health care team members, even though changes in reimbursement policies would contribute to eliminating health inequities.[22]

In addition to the historical omission of the full cadre of interprofessional health care workers, the traditional paradigms associated with the current US health care system have restricted the scope of practice of nonphysician members of the health care workforce.[23,24] These restrictive practices are most evident in professions such as nursing, in which there is significant variation in what is permissible regarding what advanced practice nurses are permitted to do.[23,24] These restrictions are not rooted in the preponderance of evidence, which shows the benefits of permitting all members of an interprofessional health care workforce (e.g., dental and oral health professionals, pharmacists, and physician assistants) to practice at the highest levels of their education, licenses, and competencies.[23,24] These restrictions often reflect "turf wars"[23] rather than health care delivery models that prioritize supporting the full interprofessional health care team with greatest demonstrated efficacy in eliminating health care inequities.

Finally, beyond the current restrictions in the scope of practice for the existing health care workforce, expansion of current roles, practice settings,

BOX 1— Contrasting Traditional Health Care With a "Bridged Model" of Public Health and Primary Care

Current Clinical Care Approach	Bridging Public Health and Clinical Care
Primarily focused on the diagnosis, treatment, and management of disease (i.e., sick-care model)	A primary care model that fully integrates social and clinical care and prioritizes wellness, prevention, and health promotion
Health care expenditures primarily allocated to costly diagnostic and treatment procedures	Equitable financial investment in primary care to address population health and wellness and health-related social needs
Health care workforce primarily consisting of clinicians (e.g., physicians, nurses, pharmacists)	Expanded definition of the health care workforce to include omitted actors (e.g., community health workers, social workers, behavioral health and addiction providers)
Scope of practice restrictions on nonphysician workforce members	All members of the health care workforce practicing at the highest levels of their education, licenses, and competencies
Clinical care with referral to health-related social needs	An integrated, interprofessional, team-based workforce with collective responsibility and leadership in the delivery of clinical and social care
Health profession training that primarily occurs in clinic settings (e.g., hospitals) and is patient focused	Health profession training that occurs across a range of settings (e.g., correctional facilities, schools, hospitals) with families in communities
Health care workforce largely not representative of the communities served	Representative and diverse health care workforce with cultural/linguistic preparedness
Delivery of services primarily within traditional clinical settings	Locational flexibility of services aligned with community needs (e.g., telehealth, home based, community-based organizations)
Episodic/sporadic clinical care delivery	Predictable, relationship-based, person-centered and whole-person care
Lack of meaningful engagement of racial and ethnically minoritized communities	Intentional engagement and alignment of the health care system with community needs built on trustworthiness, equal power, and shared decision making
A health care system that overly emphasizes cost containment and, to a lesser degree, access and quality without specific prioritization of the elimination of health care inequities and the achievement of health equity	Sustained organizational commitment to the elimination of health care inequities through implementation of systemic and structural changes within the health care system that prioritize health equity on par with addressing access, quality, and cost containment

and care delivery processes is needed.[22] A more effective interprofessional workforce will increasingly require that we consider alternative settings where care can be provided—homes, via telehealth, within community-based organizations, schools, and so forth—and a team with collective responsibility and equal leadership in the provision of integrated care.[2,22–24]

A NEW VISION: BRIDGING PUBLIC HEALTH AND CLINICAL CARE

A primary health care system for the future will undoubtedly benefit from bridging the traditional aspects of public health to reimagine a more effective and robust primary health care system. In this new model of integrated care, population health is the primary goal. At the cornerstone of this integrated clinical and social primary care model is public health, which has a strong "bridge" to traditional health care service delivery. Public health provides a framework for prevention and health promotion within primary care. In addition, public health workers are accustomed to engaging with interprofessional teams across multiple levels of intervention (e.g., individuals, institutions, communities and broader societies)[17] and across diverse settings such as schools, correctional facilities, substance use treatment programs, community centers, and homes.

As noted by Baum et al., however, significant barriers such as siloed funding, resource limitations, and a lack of collective awareness and action in the integration of clinical care and public health hinder such efforts.[25] Nevertheless, a "bridged model" of primary care that draws on the clinical expertise of the primary care workforce and shifts the emphasis to prioritization of health prevention and promotion, consistent with the field of public health (Box 1), has the potential to dramatically shift the current trajectory of illness in the United States.

To achieve this goal, we need to engage health profession schools and licensing and accreditation bodies and advocate for changes in curricula and clinical experiences. Much greater emphasis will need to be placed on training the future health care workforce in communities and alongside a broad set of team members who are experienced in working together without unnecessary restrictions and under equal footing with respect to their contributions to eliminating health inequities.

Substantial challenges related to multilevel change within health care systems must be forcefully addressed to eliminate health care inequities. AJPH

CORRESPONDENCE

Correspondence should be sent to Vincent Guilamo-Ramos, PhD, MPH, LCSW, ANP-BC, PMHNP-BC, Institute for Policy Solutions, School of Nursing, Johns Hopkins University, 555 Pennsylvania Ave NW, Suite #450, Washington, DC 20001 (e-mail: vincentramos@jhu.edu). Reprints can be ordered at https://www.ajph.org by clicking the "Reprints" link.

PUBLICATION INFORMATION

Full Citation: Guilamo-Ramos V, Amankwah FK, Tucker-Seeley R, Jernigan VBB, Benjamin GC. Toward community-engaged health care to bridge public health with clinical care. *Am J Public Health*. 2024;114(12):1300–1304.

Acceptance Date: July 18, 2024.

DOI: https://www.doi.org/10.2105/AJPH.2024.307816

ORCID iD:

Georges C. Benjamin https://orcid.org/0000-0003-3453-1654

CONTRIBUTORS

V. Guilamo-Ramos contributed to the conceptualization, drafting, and editing of the article. F. K. Amankwah, R. Tucker-Seely, V. Blue Bird Jernigan, and G. C. Benjamin contributed to the conceptualization, review, and revision of the article.

ACKNOWLEDGMENTS

This research was sponsored by the National Institutes of Health (NIH) and the Agency for Healthcare Research and Quality (AHRQ).

We acknowledge the essential contributions of the members of the Committee on Unequal Treatment Revisited: The Current State of Racial and Ethnic Disparities in Health Care.

Note. The funders of the report, NIH and AHRQ, had no role in the preparation, review, or approval of this article or the decision to submit the article for publication.

CONFLICTS OF INTEREST

V. Guilamo-Ramos is a member of the National Advisory Council for Nursing Research as of May 2024. The views expressed in this manuscript are not a reflection of the National Institute of Nursing Research (NINR) or NIH. Neither NINR nor NIH played a role in the preparation, review, or approval of this *AJPH* manuscript, or the decision to submit the manuscript for publication. The coauthors certify that they have no affiliations with or involvement in any organization or entity with any financial or nonfinancial interest in the subject matter or materials discussed in this article.

REFERENCES

1. Institute of Medicine. *Unequal Treatment: Confronting Racial and Ethnic Disparities in Health Care.* Washington, DC: National Academies Press; 2003.
2. National Academies of Sciences, Engineering, and Medicine. *Ending Unequal Treatment: Strategies to Achieve Equitable Health Care and Optimal Health for All.* Washington, DC: National Academies Press; 2024.
3. Schneider EC, Shah A, Doty MM, Tikkanen R, Fields K, Williams RD II. Health care in the US compared to other high-income countries. Available at: https://www.commonwealthfund.org/publications/fund-reports/2021/aug/mirror-mirror-2021-reflecting-poorly. Accessed June 28, 2024.
4. Fiore JA, Madison AJ, Poisal JA, et al. National health expenditure projections, 2023–32: payer trends diverge as pandemic-related policies fade. *Health Aff (Millwood).* 2024;43(7):910–921. https://doi.org/10.1377/hlthaff.2024.00469
5. Stange KC, Miller WL, Etz RS. The role of primary care in improving population health. *Milbank Q.* 2023;101(suppl 1):795–840. https://doi.org/10.1111/1468-0009.12638
6. Lantz PM, Goldberg DS, Gollust SE. The perils of medicalization for population health and health equity. *Milbank Q.* 2023;101(suppl 1):61–82. https://doi.org/10.1111/1468-0009.12619
7. Boersma P, Black LI, Ward BW. Prevalence of multiple chronic conditions among US adults, 2018. *Prev Chronic Dis.* 2020;17:200130. https://doi.org/10.5888/pcd17.200130
8. Arias E, Tejada-Vera B, Kochanek KD, Ahmad FB. Provisional life expectancy estimates for 2021. Available at: https://stacks.cdc.gov/view/cdc/118999. Accessed June 28, 2024.
9. National Indian Health Board. Advancing health equity through the federal trust responsibility: full mandatory funding for the Indian Health Service and strengthening nation-to-nation relationships. Available at: https://www.nihb.org/docs/09072022/FY%202024%20Tribal%20Budget%20Formulation%20Workgroup%20Recommendations.pdf. Accessed June 28, 2024.
10. Centers for Disease Control and Prevention. Health and economic costs of chronic diseases. Available at: https://www.cdc.gov/chronicdisease/about/costs/index.htm. Accessed June 28, 2024.
11. Wang L, Si L, Cocker F, Palmer AJ, Sanderson K. A systematic review of cost-of-illness studies of multimorbidity. *Appl Health Econ Health Policy.* 2018;16(1):15–29. https://doi.org/10.1007/s40258-017-0346-6
12. LaVeist TA, Pérez-Stable EJ, Richard P, et al. The economic burden of racial, ethnic, and educational health inequities in the US. *JAMA.* 2023;329(19):1682–1692. https://doi.org/10.1001/jama.2023.5965
13. Chuang E, Safaeinili N. Addressing social needs in clinical settings: implementation and impact on health care utilization, costs, and integration of care. *Annu Rev Public Health.* 2023;45:443–464. https://doi.org/10.1146/annurev-publhealth-061022-050026
14. Agonafer EP, Carson SL, Nunez V, et al. Community-based organizations' perspectives on improving health and social service integration. *BMC Public Health.* 2021;21(1):452. https://doi.org/10.1186/s12889-021-10449-w
15. Dickman SL, Himmelstein DU, Woolhandler S. Inequality and the health-care system in the USA. *Lancet.* 2017;389(10077):1431–1441. https://doi.org/10.1016/S0140-6736(17)30398-7
16. Thimm-Kaiser M, Benzekri A, Guilamo-Ramos V. Conceptualizing the mechanisms of social determinants of health: a heuristic framework to inform future directions for mitigation. *Milbank Q.* 2023;101(2):486–526. https://doi.org/10.1111/1468-0009.12642
17. Guilamo-Ramos V, Thimm-Kaiser M, Benzekri A, et al. Application of a heuristic framework for multilevel interventions to eliminate the impact of unjust social processes and other harmful social determinants of health. *Prev Sci.* 2024;25(suppl 3):446–458. https://doi.org/10.1007/s11121-024-01658-x
18. D'Agostino EM, Oto-Kent D, Nuño M. Paving the way for the next frontier of community-engaged research. *Am J Public Health.* 2024;114(suppl 5):S347–S349. https://doi.org/10.2105/AJPH.2024.307685
19. Mensah GA, Johnson LE. Community Engagement Alliance (CEAL): leveraging the power of communities during public health emergencies. *Am J Public Health.* 2024;114(suppl 1):S18–S21. https://doi.org/10.2105/AJPH.2023.307507
20. Guilamo-Ramos V, Thimm-Kaiser M, Benzekri A. Community-engaged mpox vaccination provides lessons for equitable health care in the United States. *Nat Med.* 2023;29(9):2160–2161. https://doi.org/10.1038/s41591-023-02447-9
21. Blue Bird Jernigan V, Peercy M, Branam D, et al. Beyond health equity: achieving wellness within American Indian and Alaska Native communities. *Am J Public Health.* 2015;105(suppl 3):S376–S379. https://doi.org/10.2105/AJPH.2014.302447
22. Noel L, Chen Q, Petruzzi LJ, et al. Interprofessional collaboration between social workers and community health workers to address health and mental health in the United States: a systematised review. *Health Soc Care Community.* 2022;30(6):e6240–e6254. https://doi.org/10.1111/hsc.14061
23. Frogner BK, Patterson DG, Skillman SM. The workforce needed to address population health. *Milbank Q.* 2023;101(suppl 1):841–865. https://doi.org/10.1111/1468-0009.12620
24. Chen AJ, Munnich EL, Parente ST, Richards MR. Provider turf wars and Medicare payment rules. *J Public Econ.* 2023;218:104812. https://doi.org/10.1016/j.jpubeco.2022.104812
25. Baum NM, Iovan S, Udow-Phillips M. Strengthening public health through primary care and public health collaboration: innovative state approaches. *J Public Health Manag Pract.* 2024;30(2):E47–E53 https://doi.org/10.1097/phh.0000000000001860

The Call for a School-Based Approach to Opioid Overdose Prevention

Jessica B. Calihan, MD, MS, Brittany L. Carney, DNP, FNP-BC, Deb M. Schmill, BS, and Sarah M. Bagley, MD, MSc

ABOUT THE AUTHORS

Jessica B. Calihan and Sarah M. Bagley are with the Division of Health Services Research, Department of Pediatrics, Chobanian & Avedisian School of Medicine and Boston Medical Center Boston, Boston, MA. Brittany L. Carney and Sarah M. Bagley are with the Section of General Internal Medicine, Department of Medicine, Boston University Chobanian & Avedisian School of Medicine, Boston, MA. Brittany L. Carney is also with the Grayken Center for Addiction Training and Technical Assistance & Department of Pediatrics, Adolescent Medicine, Boston Medical Center, Boston, MA. Deb M. Schmill is with the Becca Schmill Foundation, Needham, MA.

Drug overdose is the third leading cause of death among children and adolescents in the United States.[1] Although youth substance use, including opioid use, decreased in recent decades, there was a 121% increase in adolescent overdose deaths from 2010 to 2021.[2,3] This dramatic increase is driven by a toxic drug supply, with synthetically manufactured opioids like fentanyl contributing to the majority of adolescent deaths.[2,4] Among youths who died from an overdose from 2019 to 2021, 65% did not have a history of opioid use, 89% had never received substance use disorder treatment, and naloxone was used only 33% of the time.[4] These trends emphasize the inadequacy of current responses to adolescent overdose. In the current context, adolescent substance use is increasingly risky, and it is insufficient to focus only on primary prevention strategies. It is clear that we need an urgent public health strategy to provide youths with overdose prevention education and information about how to use naloxone. Although this article emphasizes adolescent-focused public health strategies, reducing adolescent opioid overdose deaths will also require engaging families, school staff, providers, and other adults who care for youths.

An efficacious prevention strategy would universally teach individuals how to recognize and respond to an overdose with naloxone administration, which is foundational to opioid overdose response. Naloxone is an opioid antagonist and Food and Drug Administration–approved opioid overdose reversal medication. Two versions (4 mg and 3 mg nasal sprays) were approved for over-the-counter sale in 2023.[5] Public health strategies to improve naloxone utilization, including state laws providing access without a prescription (before naloxone became over the counter) and provision of civil liability protection to laypeople administering naloxone, have helped decrease opioid overdose mortality and have not been associated with an increase in nonmedical opioid use by adolescents or adults.[6,7] However, adult-focused implementation strategies to improve access to naloxone are not reaching youths. Per capita dispensing of naloxone remains lowest among those aged birth to 19 years,[8] and a review of Centers for Disease Control and Prevention 2019–2021 data found that naloxone was not administered in 70% of fatal overdoses in those aged 10 to 19 years despite the presence of a potential bystander in 67% of the cases.[4]

Overdose education with naloxone distribution (OEND) is a proven public health strategy that reduces opioid overdose deaths in adults and may be one way to improve youth naloxone access.[9] However, there are currently limited models for implementing OEND content in youth-focused and accessible settings. Schools offer public health education on a number of youth-specific risk behaviors. Naloxone implementation in schools offers an opportunity for universal youth education and prevention of fatal overdose in a space where youths spend substantial time. An open letter published by the US Department of Education and Office of National Drug Control Policy in October 2023 called for schools to develop plans to educate students and personnel on overdose response, noting that "there is no time to waste when responding to an overdose, and it is critical that youth and school personnel can access naloxone on school grounds during and after school."[10–13] However, there are limited evidence-based interventions to educate school personnel and students on overdose prevention, recognition, and intervention.

In this essay, we review barriers to youth naloxone access, describe legislative efforts to improve access in schools, and discuss potential opportunities for youth-focused opioid overdose prevention education.

AJPH December 2024, Vol. 114, No. 12

BARRIERS TO YOUTH NALOXONE ACCESS

Adolescent access to naloxone is likely influenced by inadequate youth overdose education, pharmacy barriers, insufficient provider prescribing, limited data on adolescent overdose risk factors, and stigma surrounding adolescent use. As a result of insufficient adolescent education, college students report limited knowledge of naloxone use (30%) and administration (14%).[14]

Pharmacy barriers include the high cost of over-the-counter naloxone and prevalent incorrect pharmacist assumptions about minimum age requirements.[15] Adolescents also worry about pharmacist or provider judgment, feel embarrassed, and misunderstand the need for parental consent when accessing stigmatized medications.[16]

Pediatric providers are also not meeting the needs of youth naloxone prescribing. Insufficient pediatrician and provider education persists, which may limit naloxone prescribing and further contribute to poor adolescent naloxone access.[17] Although pediatricians feel that overdose prevention is their responsibility and they can identify at-risk youths, very few pediatric trainees (10%) report ever prescribing naloxone, and only 14% of pediatric emergency room physicians report providing naloxone after an opioid-related visit.[17,18] Prescribing patterns are likely influenced by limited naloxone knowledge, lack of education on addressing overdose risk with patients, and provider stigma around who is at risk for overdose.[17]

Recent data show that most adolescents who died of an overdose had no history of an opioid use disorder. This suggests a need to reconceptualize prior data identifying youth overdose risk factors such as injection drug use, prior opioid use, and sedative use as risk factors for youth opioid overdose. If youths are overdosing on fentanyl-contaminated pills the first time that they try substances, focusing on improving naloxone distribution to youths already known to use substances will be insufficient in preventing overdose deaths.

LEGISLATIVE EFFORTS TO IMPROVE NALOXONE ACCESS IN SCHOOLS

Schools offer a promising opportunity to provide universal prevention through OEND in a setting where many youths already receive education on public health topics and risk behaviors. Making naloxone available in the case of an emergency is an important component of such a strategy. US schools have adopted response programs for a range of potentially fatal emergencies, including opioid overdose. As of 2017, 17 states required the installation of automated external defibrillators for use in sudden cardiac arrest, and as of 2018, all 50 states and the District of Columbia enacted laws facilitating the use of undesignated epinephrine in the case of anaphylaxis.[19] Currently 36 states allow schools or school employees to store, possess, or administer naloxone on school campuses.[20] However, requirements differ by state; only two states (Illinois and Rhode Island) require all private and public schools (kindergarten to 12th grade) to stock opioid antagonists, whereas Arkansas, Maryland, Minnesota, New Jersey, and Oregon require all public high schools to stock opioid antagonists.[20]

Access to naloxone in US schools may improve with the passage of the recently proposed School Access to Naloxone Act of 2023 (S.2946, H.R.3065) or the proposed Stop Overdose in Schools Act (H.R.5652), which would incentivize schools to maintain opioid overdose reversal agents that can be administered by trained personnel under civil liability protection law.[11,12,21] The Helping Educators Respond to Overdoses (HERO) Act (H.R.6251) would establish grants to fund the development and implementation of overdose prevention curricula for students and community members in addition to the purchase of opioid overdose reversal agents.[13] The School Access to Naloxone Act of 2023 is supported by the National Association of School Nurses, which recommends that opioid overdose management plans be incorporated into school emergency preparedness and response plans,[22] and by the American College Health Association, which recommends that college health centers be prepared to respond to an opioid overdose and add naloxone to emergency kits.[23]

YOUTH-FOCUSED OVERDOSE PREVENTION EDUCATION

Improving naloxone availability and training in schools is a promising development, with the potential to save lives. However, the School Access to Naloxone Act misses an opportunity to improve universal prevention of overdose deaths outside of school by not requiring youth overdose education. Classroom-based interventions are a common primary substance use prevention strategy, yet existing programs do not generally incorporate overdose education, including use of naloxone. As naloxone is potentially introduced into more schools, there is an urgent need to implement overdose prevention curricula in schools. Although the HERO Act recognizes this need, it does not emphasize the equally urgent need to develop outcome measures and evaluate curricula to ensure that youths are receiving efficacious and youth-focused messages. Previously, non-evidence-based substance use prevention curricula (e.g., Project DARE) were widely adopted in US schools and received substantial government support despite an absence of proven efficacy.[24] Curricula should present evidence about opioids, overdose risk, and appropriate response while addressing common myths—for example, that topical fentanyl exposure causes overdose, or that fentanyl is present in nicotine or cannabis vapes—that may make youths reluctant to respond and may perpetuate stigma related to drug use.[25]

Opioid overdose education and prevention curricula currently implemented in limited high school settings include Safety First, which uses thirteen 55-minute sessions to discuss signs of problematic substance use, harm reduction strategies, and overdose response, and the Rx for Addiction and Medication Safety program, which includes two to three interactive education sessions on opioid safety, misuse, and overdose.[26,27] In pilot studies of participating ninth graders, these curricula are associated with improved confidence and skills in understanding harm reduction strategies, identifying overdose, utilizing naloxone, and educating friends and families on opioid overdose response.[26,27] Neither study evaluated postintervention use of naloxone.

On college campuses, interventions combining free naloxone distribution with naloxone education are well-received by students and are associated with improved knowledge of opioid overdose risks and readiness to respond to an overdose. They are also linked to increased access to naloxone on campus, which can lead to successful overdose reversals.[28,29] These college programs are currently opt-in, and it is unknown how effectively they could be universally applied in a high school setting.

Opioid overdose curricula have also been piloted in juvenile detention centers, where youths may be at particularly high risk of overdose.[30] In these settings, the combination of overdose response education and distribution of naloxone kits on release was associated with increased naloxone knowledge, confidence managing an opioid overdose, and, in one evaluation of postrelease follow-up, willingness to share knowledge.[30,31] Youths engaged in these interventions did report concerns about legal repercussions of overdose response (e.g., arrest for being at the scene of opioid use), suggesting that education on civil liability protections when appropriate may improve readiness to respond.[31] Despite these promising results, it is unknown how applicable these interventions may be in high school settings, where youths may have less familiarity with overdose preintervention.

CONCLUSION

Adolescents are dying at an increasing rate from opioid overdose. Most of these youths have no history of documented opioid use or treatment of other substance use disorders. Reliance on overdose strategies targeting youths with previously described overdose risk factors such as injection drug use or prior opioid use is insufficient. Instead, a universal public health overdose prevention strategy is needed to save lives when there is an increasingly toxic drug supply. Overdose deaths are preventable when youths can access naloxone and overdose prevention education that is evidence-based and acceptable to youths. Yet public health efforts to expand naloxone access focused on adults and patients with a history of opioid use have not addressed gaps in provider knowledge, pharmacy access, and understanding of overdose risk factors that limit youth access. There is a desperate need for new public health strategies targeting youths to prevent further adolescent deaths.

The School Access to Naloxone Act of 2023 and related proposed legislation are a promising opportunity to improve naloxone availability for youths. However, to universally address overdose risk and prevent fatal overdoses, we need evidence-based naloxone education for youths that can be implemented in diverse school settings alongside accessible naloxone. Promising studies suggest that interactive, case-based interventions improve youth knowledge of overdose risk and naloxone use, but curricula implementation remains limited. As members of the public health community, we must advocate for the inclusion of evidence-based educational interventions alongside improved naloxone access to address opioid-related risk, prevent further deaths, and improve health for all youths. AJPH

CORRESPONDENCE

Correspondence should be sent to Jessica B. Calihan, 801 Albany St, Boston, MA 02119 (e-mail: jessica.calihan@bmc.org). Reprints can be ordered at https://www.ajph.org by clicking the "Reprints" link.

PUBLICATION INFORMATION

Full Citation: Calihan JB, Carney BL, Schmill DM, Bagley SM. The call for a school-based approach to opioid overdose prevention. *Am J Public Health.* 2024;114(12):1305–1308.

Acceptance Date: August 11, 2024.

DOI: https://doi.org/10.2105/AJPH.2024.307849

ORCID iDs:
Jessica B. Calihan https://orcid.org/0000-0003-4495-5995

Brittany L. Carney https://orcid.org/0009-0008-1195-8026

CONTRIBUTORS

J. B. Calihan and S. M. Bagley conceptualized the article's purpose, J. B. Calihan wrote the preliminary draft, and all authors contributed to manuscript revisions and approved the final version.

CONFLICTS OF INTEREST

The authors have no conflicts of interest to report.

REFERENCES

1. Goldstick JE, Cunningham RM, Carter PM. Current causes of death in children and adolescents in the United States. *N Engl J Med.* 2022;386(20):1955–1956. https://doi.org/10.1056/NEJMc2201761
2. Friedman J, Godvin M, Shover CL, Gone JP, Hansen H, Schriger DL. Trends in drug overdose deaths among US adolescents, January 2010 to June 2021. *JAMA.* 2022;327(14):1398–1400. https://doi.org/10.1001/jama.2022.2847
3. Miech RA, Johnston LD, Patrick ME, O'Malley PM, Bachman JG. National survey results on drug use, 1975–2023: overview and detailed results for secondary school students. National Institute on Drug Abuse, National Institutes of Health. 2023. Available at: https://monitoringthefuture.org/wp-content/uploads/2023/12/mtf2023.pdf. Accessed January 2, 2024.
4. Tanz LJ. Drug overdose deaths among persons aged 10–19 years—United States, July 2019–December 2021. *MMWR Morb Mortal Wkly Rep.* 2022;71(50):1576–1582. https://doi.org/10.15585/mmwr.mm7150a2
5. US Food and Drug Administration. FDA approves second over-the-counter naloxone nasal spray product. August 1, 2023. Available at: https://www.fda.gov/news-events/press-announcements/fda-approves-second-over-counter-naloxone-nasal-spray-product. Accessed July 17, 2024.
6. McClellan C, Lambdin BH, Ali MM, et al. Opioid-overdose laws association with opioid use and overdose mortality. *Addict Behav.* 2018;86:90–95. https://doi.org/10.1016/j.addbeh.2018.03.014
7. Bruzelius E, Cerda M, Davis CS, et al. Naloxone expansion is not associated with increases in adolescent heroin use and injection drug use: evidence from 44 US states. *Int J Drug Policy.* 2023;114:103980. https://doi.org/10.1016/j.drugpo.2023.103980
8. Guy GP, Haegerich TM, Evans ME, Losby JL, Young R, Jones CM. Vital signs: pharmacy-based naloxone dispensing—United States, 2012–2018. *MMWR Morb Mortal Wkly Rep.* 2019;68(31):679–686. https://doi.org/10.15585/mmwr.mm6831e1
9. Walley AY, Xuan Z, Hackman HH, et al. Opioid overdose rates and implementation of overdose education and nasal naloxone distribution in Massachusetts: interrupted time series analysis. *BMJ.* 2013;346:f174. https://doi.org/10.1136/bmj.f174
10. Cardona MA, Gupta R. Letter to schools. October 30, 2023. Available at: https://www.whitehouse.gov/wp-content/uploads/2023/10/Letter-to-Schools.pdf. Accessed November 27, 2023.
11. Merkley J. S2946—School Access to Naloxone Act of 2023. 2023. Available at: https://www.congress.gov/bill/118th-congress/senate-bill/2946. Accessed November 27, 2023.
12. Phillips D. HR3065—School Access to Naloxone Act of 2023. 2023. Available at: https://www.congress.gov/bill/118th-congress/house-bill/3065. Accessed July 21, 2024.
13. Schiff AB. HR6251—Helping Educators Respond to Overdoses Act. 2023. Available at: https://www.congress.gov/bill/118th-congress/house-bill/6251/text. Accessed July 21, 2024.
14. Freibott CE, Vest N, Stein MD, Lipson SK. Opioid overdose knowledge among adolescents and young adults. *JAMA Pediatr.* 2024;178(6):618–620. https://doi.org/10.1001/jamapediatrics.2024.0561
15. Jimenez DE, Singer MR, Adesman A. Availability of naloxone in pharmacies and knowledge of pharmacy staff regarding dispensing naloxone to younger adolescents. *J Adolesc Health.* 2019;65(5):698–701. https://doi.org/10.1016/j.jadohealth.2019.07.009
16. Williams BN, Jauk VC, Szychowski JM, Arbuckle JL. Adolescent emergency contraception usage, knowledge, and perception. *Contraception.* 2021;103(5):361–366. https://doi.org/10.1016/j.contraception.2021.01.003
17. Wilson JD, Berk J, Adger H, Feldman L. Identifying missed clinical opportunities in delivery of overdose prevention and naloxone prescription to adolescents using opioids. *J Adolesc Health.* 2018;63(2):245–248. https://doi.org/10.1016/j.jadohealth.2018.05.011
18. Hoch AM, Schoenberger SF, Boyle TP, Hadland SE, Gai MJ, Bagley SM. Attitudes and training related to substance use in pediatric emergency departments. *Addict Sci Clin Pract.* 2022;17(1):59. https://doi.org/10.1186/s13722-022-00339-w
19. Volerman A, Brindley C, Amerson N, Pressley T, Woolverton N. A national review of state laws for stock epinephrine in schools. *J Sch Health.* 2022;92(2):209–222. https://doi.org/10.1111/josh.13119
20. Legislative Analysis and Public Policy Association. Opioid antagonist access: summary of state laws. 2023. Available at: https://legislativeanalysis.org/wp-content/uploads/2023/10/Opioid-Antagonist-Access-Summary-of-State-Laws.pdf. Accessed November 1, 2023.
21. Newhouse D. Stop Overdose in Schools Act. 2023. Available at: https://www.congress.gov/bill/118th-congress/house-bill/5652/related-bills. Accessed July 21, 2024.
22. Levasseur S, Nelson L, Crowe D, Major KE. Naloxone in the school setting: position statement. *Natl Assoc Sch Nurses.* 2016;31(2):119–120. https://doi.org/10.1177/1942602X15622637
23. American College Health Association. ACHA guidelines: opioid prescribing in college health. October 2016. Available at: https://www.acha.org/resource/opioid-prescribing-in-college-health. Accessed November 26, 2023.
24. Ennett ST, Tobler NS, Ringwalt CL, Flewelling RL. How effective is drug abuse resistance education? A meta-analysis of Project DARE outcome evaluations. *Am J Public Health.* 1994;84(9):1394–1401. https://doi.org/10.2105/AJPH.84.9.1394
25. Del Pozo B, Rich JD, Carroll JJ. Reports of accidental fentanyl overdose among police in the field: toward correcting a harmful culture-bound syndrome. *Int J Drug Policy.* 2022;100:103520. https://doi.org/10.1016/j.drugpo.2021.103520
26. Fischer NR. School-based harm reduction with adolescents: a pilot study. *Subst Abuse Treat Prev Policy.* 2022;17(1):79. https://doi.org/10.1186/s13011-022-00502-1
27. Patry E, Bratberg JP, Buchanan A, Paiva AL, Balestrieri S, Matson KL. Rx for Addiction and Medication Safety: an evaluation of teen education for opioid misuse prevention. *Res Social Adm Pharm.* 2019;15(8):917–924. https://doi.org/10.1016/j.sapharm.2018.07.006
28. Hill LG, Holleran Steiker LK, Mazin L, Kinzly ML. Implementation of a collaborative model for opioid overdose prevention on campus. *J Am Coll Health.* 2020;68(3):223–226. https://doi.org/10.1080/07448481.2018.1549049
29. Doughty B, Young S, Eggleston W. Assessment of a comprehensive naloxone education program's impact on community member knowledge and attitudes on a college campus. *J Am Coll Health.* 2022;70(5):1332–1335. https://doi.org/10.1080/07448481.2020.1807992
30. Chambers S, Baca M, Navrotskaya E, et al. Pilot study of an overdose first aid program in juvenile detention. *Health Promot Pract.* 2021;22(5):638–640. https://doi.org/10.1177/1524839920950028
31. Hammond A, Obrecht J, Odunuyi O, Magloire P, Walsh S. Naloxone knowledge and attitudes of juvenile residents in a detention setting. *J Correct Health Care.* 2022;28(3):148–154. https://doi.org/10.1089/jchc.20.10.0096

Challenges and Opportunities for Wastewater Monitoring of Influenza Viruses During the Multistate Outbreak of Highly Pathogenic Avian Influenza A(H5N1) Virus in Dairy Cattle and Poultry

Margaret A. Honein, PhD, Sonja J. Olsen, PhD, Daniel B. Jernigan, MD, and Demetre C. Daskalakis, MD

ABOUT THE AUTHORS

Margaret A. Honein and Daniel B. Jernigan are with the National Center for Emerging and Zoonotic Infectious Diseases, Centers for Disease Control and Prevention (CDC), Atlanta, GA. Sonja J. Olsen and Demetre C. Daskalakis are with the National Center for Immunization and Respiratory Diseases, CDC.

The Centers for Disease Control and Prevention (CDC) began wastewater monitoring in September 2020 to provide additional information to health care providers and the public on the level of transmission of severe acute respiratory syndrome coronavirus 2 (SARS-CoV-2), the virus that causes COVID-19, and to inform public health actions.[1] This wastewater monitoring rapidly grew from a small number of states to a system in all 50 states that includes approximately 40% of the US population. Wastewater monitoring complements traditional clinical monitoring systems by detecting viruses being shed from infected individuals that might otherwise be missed; infections from asymptomatic individuals and those who do not seek or have access to clinical testing or care might be captured in wastewater-monitoring data from a given sewershed.[2]

Wastewater-monitoring data have been particularly valuable for managing COVID-19 because of the high rate of asymptomatic infections in humans contributing to SARS-CoV-2 transmission. Use of SARS-CoV-2 data from wastewater testing has been linked to successful public health actions, such as increasing uptake of vaccines through positioning of and communication about vaccination clinics.[3,4] The CDC and other public health and academic partners have expanded wastewater monitoring in the United States and globally to other pathogens, including influenza A viruses.[5–9] Although both influenza viruses and coronaviruses have zoonotic hosts, the animal hosts for SARS-CoV-2 appear significantly less likely to contribute to wastewater than do the dairy cattle and milk that are central to the current outbreak of highly pathogenic avian influenza (HPAI) A(H5N1) virus in animals.[10]

In the context of the current zoonotic outbreak of HPAI A(H5N1) virus in livestock, the CDC is monitoring for human infections using multiple systems, including public health laboratory testing to track influenza viruses such as novel viruses, trends in clinical laboratory data for influenza, and emergency department visits potentially associated with influenza.[11] There have been 14 instances of avian influenza A(H5) virus infection in people in the United States since 2022, 13 of which occurred between January and August 2024; these have been among people exposed to either infected poultry or infected dairy cattle. To use wastewater monitoring to complement traditional monitoring systems, it is urgent to better understand the meaning of influenza A virus levels and the H5 subtype in wastewater to inform public health emergency response action.

CURRENT STATUS OF WASTEWATER TESTING

Influenza A virus testing is being conducted on samples from more than 700 wastewater sites across 48 states, with testing occurring one to three times per week and data reported to CDC on a weekly basis. The CDC began publicly reporting wastewater data for influenza A viruses in May 2024 with an interim measure comparing the current

AJPH December 2024, Vol. 114, No. 12

level of influenza A virus in each wastewater site to the levels observed in the same wastewater site from October 1, 2023, to March 2, 2024.[12] This comparison period aligns with the human influenza season period before the detection of HPAI A(H5N1) virus in dairy cattle. This approach was implemented because the initial detections of influenza A(H5) virus subtype in wastewater coincided with large influenza A virus spikes occurring toward the end of the influenza season.[13]

By focusing on areas with unusually high influenza virus levels in wastewater (≥ 80th percentile) during a time when influenza infections were expected to be lower or decreasing, public health officials could quickly investigate the high influenza A virus levels. However, this interim measure limited the number of sites with sufficient data for analysis because it restricted analyses to sites that had begun testing for influenza A virus no later than October 1, 2023. Although data were submitted for more than 700 sites each week, less than half of the sites had sufficient data for analysis by this method because of the start date for their testing, the timeliness of data submission, or other missing information.

As we approach fall 2024, when seasonal influenza will begin to circulate more widely, the CDC is evaluating and validating an updated approach to monitoring influenza virus levels in wastewater over time in a manner that is similar to the wastewater viral activity measure used for SARS-CoV-2. In November 2023, the CDC initiated monitoring SARS-CoV-2 using the wastewater viral activity level, which allows aggregating data at the state, regional, and national levels rather than comparing each site's data only to its own previous data.[14] A similar approach to influenza A virus will allow clearer communication to the public by providing data on influenza levels at the state and national levels.

CHALLENGES WITH WASTEWATER TESTING

Testing for influenza A viruses in wastewater is challenging for a number of reasons, and the complexity has increased with the emergence of the HPAI A(H5N1) virus outbreak in dairy cattle.[15,16] First, among those infected with influenza A virus, the virus might only be intermittently shed in feces, and there are limited data on viral concentrations in feces and urine.[17] Second, influenza A viruses infect humans but also are commonly found in animals and wild birds, such as waterfowl, which are the natural reservoir. Most wastewater systems in the United States are closed systems; however, open or combined wastewater systems receive storm water runoff, which could include inputs from wild birds. Some closed systems might also periodically receive inputs from sources accessible to wild birds.

Third, wastewater systems have a variety of inputs in addition to household sources (e.g., toilet, sink, and shower water). Some wastewater systems receive large volumes of input from milk- or meat-processing plants, inputs from poultry farms, and in some cases inputs from other agricultural sources that contain livestock waste. Current techniques do not allow determination of whether the source of the influenza A virus or subtype in wastewater is from an animal or a human source. Studies have shown that cattle have avian-specific receptors in both mammary and respiratory tissue and that the H5 virus can be found in very high levels in unpasteurized milk and in the lungs, muscle, and udder tissue.[18] Detection of avian influenza A(H5) virus in wastewater is an important surveillance indicator and likely provides an indirect measure of the outbreak of HPAI A(H5N1) virus in dairy cattle in the United States, but it but does not provide clarity on whether any human infections are contributing viral particles.

Fourth, we do not know how much avian influenza A(H5) virus is needed to result in a positive H5 subtype detection in a wastewater system (i.e., sensitivity) and how that might vary by the size of the population served by a single sewershed, which can range from thousands to millions. And fifth, differences in laboratory approaches and reporting approaches can complicate interpretation[19]; the CDC is currently validating an influenza A H5 subtype molecular detection assay for use in wastewater with the intention of sharing the protocol and recommending its use as a reference standard testing assay before the start of the 2024/2025 influenza season.

Despite these challenges, wastewater monitoring for influenza A virus and H5 subtype and close coordination with local public health officials to better understand the likely sources of influenza A(H5) virus in wastewater can help refine methods for use in the upcoming influenza season. For example, detection of H5 in wastewater could trigger additional monitoring or testing of animals, milk, or humans.

WASTEWATER TESTING FOR HPAI A(H5N1)

A report released recently in the CDC's *Morbidity and Mortality Weekly Report* highlights the findings and follow-up public health investigations for high levels of influenza A virus and H5 subtype detection in wastewater.[20] The H5 testing in wastewater used a quantitative test, but public health investigations were triggered by any qualitative detection of H5 in wastewater.[13]

In three out of four states with detections of high levels of influenza A virus in wastewater, there were consistent findings from other human clinical influenza-monitoring systems reflecting late seasonal influenza epidemic activity in certain communities. There was no evidence of avian influenza (HPAI) A(H5N1) virus detected in people in the states with high influenza A virus levels in wastewater. By contrast, eight of nine states with HPAI A(H5) virus detections in wastewater occurred in states with reported HPAI A(H5N1) virus–infected herds.

And, despite H5 testing of wastewater occurring in 41 states, only nine states had one or more sites with an H5 detection during the nine-week period of the investigations with a high correlation between reported infected herds and detection of H5 in wastewater. States with H5 detections in wastewater identified potential contributing sources of animal inputs, including dairies or milk-processing plants, meat-processing plants, and other sources of agricultural inputs.

Some processing sites received and processed milk or meat products from outside their state, further complicating the interpretation. Testing specific areas in a sewer network (subsewershed testing) following initial detection of influenza A(H5) virus in wastewater supported the hypothesis of milk-processing plants contributing to these detections.[13] Review of existing human surveillance system data in jurisdictions with H5 detections in wastewater did not identify unusual human influenza activity, providing further evidence that these H5 detections were likely of animal origin.

LESSONS LEARNED AND PLANNING

The current outbreak of HPAI A(H5N1) virus in dairy cattle, poultry, and other animals as well as human cases identified among those with exposure to infected animals requires a One Health approach to monitor and protect human and animal health, and wastewater monitoring can be an important additional approach in this endeavor.[21]

Wastewater monitoring is a relatively new public health tool that can complement our existing health-monitoring systems to help us better track infectious diseases and guide public health actions, such as alerting clinicians about viruses circulating in the community, positioning and increasing uptake of vaccines, and alerting the public of periods of increased risk and consideration for taking personal protective measures. It provides valuable data on virus levels at the community level, even when individuals may not have symptoms or seek clinical testing, and therefore is not limited to detecting the more severe cases that require medical attention. However, wastewater monitoring is not a one-size-fits-all solution, and the value of wastewater monitoring in addition to other health-monitoring systems will depend on the jurisdiction and the specific disease to be monitored, including the following:

1. the strength and coverage of other monitoring systems;
2. the proportion of infected individuals who are asymptomatic, with wastewater monitoring having added importance in detecting asymptomatic infections given those individuals are unlikely to be seen in health care settings or tested, and the relative proportion of transmission accounted for by asymptomatic versus symptomatic individuals as well as the proportion of symptomatic individuals who do not seek health care or receive testing;
3. the role of animal reservoirs and animal product inputs to sewersheds and future laboratory techniques that might allow public health officials to distinguish human from animal sources in wastewater;
4. gaps in available information (e.g., likely zoonotic sources that have not been tested) on the state of an outbreak that can be at least partially addressed with findings from wastewater testing; and
5. the distribution of wastewater-monitoring sites in areas relevant to the pathogen being addressed.

For the current outbreak of HPAI A(H5N1) virus in dairy cattle, the consideration of these factors will vary widely among jurisdictions and likely among different areas in a jurisdiction. Monitoring for increases in influenza A virus and H5 subtype detections during times of low seasonal influenza activity, such as the summer months, can help improve planning for how to use wastewater testing efficiently with limited resources during the respiratory illness season. This approach also helps fill in critical information gaps that could slow our response to the ongoing threat from HPAI A(H5N1) viruses.

To ensure an effective wastewater-monitoring system that informs public health actions during the upcoming fall through winter respiratory illness season, it is important to incorporate the following components: (1) testing wastewater for influenza A virus and subtypes: this will facilitate detection and monitoring of different influenza viruses circulating in the human or animal population, providing insights into disease dynamics; (2) deployment of wastewater testing in high priority locations: by strategically focusing health-monitoring resources on areas with a higher risk of disease transmission or where outbreaks in people may be more likely to occur (e.g., areas with identified infected dairy cattle herds or poultry farms), we can obtain targeted data that reflect broader trends and help us prioritize public health actions; and (3) timely data integration to address knowledge gaps: wastewater monitoring can provide additional insights into disease patterns and transmission dynamics by including those who are not tested or seen in a health care setting, allowing us to track changes in viral activity and fill information gaps that may exist in monitoring systems that rely on individuals seeking and having access to care.

By incorporating these elements into national wastewater monitoring, we can improve our ability to monitor respiratory illnesses, inform public health actions, and prepare for and respond to future outbreaks. AJPH

CORRESPONDENCE

Correspondence should be sent to Margaret A. Honein, PhD, MPH, Director, Division of Infectious Disease Readiness and Innovation, National Center for Emerging and Zoonotic Infectious Diseases, CDC, 1600 Clifton Rd NE, Mailstop H-24-11, Atlanta, GA 30329 (e-mail: mhonein@cdc.gov). Reprints can be ordered at https://www.ajph.org by clicking the "Reprints" link.

PUBLICATION INFORMATION

Full Citation: Honein MA, Olsen SJ, Jernigan DB, Daskalakis DC. Challenges and opportunities for wastewater monitoring of influenza viruses during the multistate outbreak of highly pathogenic avian influenza A(H5N1) virus in dairy cattle and poultry. *Am J Public Health*. 2024;114(12): 1309–1312.

Acceptance Date: August 27, 2024.

DOI: https://doi.org/10.2105/AJPH.2024.307860

ORCID iDs:

Margaret A. Honein https://orcid.org/0000-0002-1523-7815

Sonja J. Olsen https://orcid.org/0000-0002-8983-1913

Daniel B. Jernigan https://orcid.org/0000-0002-0653-2433

CONTRIBUTORS

The authors contributed equally to this editorial.

ACKNOWLEDGMENTS

We thank Matthew Biggerstaff, Jonathan Yoder, Amy Kirby, and Nicole Fehrenbach for their helpful insights and suggestions.

This editorial is a coordinated release with the Centers for Disease Control and Prevention's Morbidity and Mortality Weekly Report found here: https://www.cdc.gov/mmwr/volumes/73/wr/mm7337a1.htm?s_cid=mm7337a1_w

Note. The findings and conclusions in this editorial are those of the authors and do not necessarily represent the views of the Centers for Disease Control and Prevention.

CONFLICTS OF INTEREST

The authors have no conflicts of interest to declare.

REFERENCES

1. Adams C, Bias M, Welsh RM, et al. The National Wastewater Surveillance System (NWSS): from inception to widespread coverage, 2020–2022, United States. *Sci Total Environ.* 2024;924:171566. https://doi.org/10.1016/j.scitotenv.2024.171566
2. Kotlarz N, Holcomb DA, Tanvir Pasha ABM, et al. Timing and trends for municipal wastewater, lab-confirmed case, and syndromic case surveillance of COVID-19 in Raleigh, North Carolina. *Am J Public Health.* 2023;113(1):79–88. https://doi.org/10.2105/AJPH.2022.307108
3. Alonso C, Keppard B, Bates S, Cortez D, Amaya F, Dinakar K. The Chelsea Project: turning research and wastewater surveillance on COVID-19 into health equity action, Massachusetts, 2020–2021. *Am J Public Health.* 2023;113(6):627–630. https://doi.org/10.2105/AJPH.2023.307253
4. Centers for Disease Control and Prevention. Notes from the field: the National Wastewater Surveillance System's Centers of Excellence contributions to public health action during the respiratory virus season—four US jurisdictions, 2022–23. *MMWR Morb Mortal Wkly Rep.* 2023;72(48):1309–1312. https://doi.org/10.15585/mmwr.mm7248a4
5. Lehto KM, Lansivaara A, Hyder R, et al. Wastewater-based surveillance is an efficient monitoring tool for tracking influenza A in the community. *Water Res.* 2024;257:121650. https://doi.org/10.1016/j.watres.2024.121650
6. Centers for Disease Control and Prevention. Wastewater surveillance data as a complement to emergency department visit data for tracking incidence of influenza A and respiratory syncytial virus—Wisconsin, August 2022–March 2023. *MMWR Morb Mortal Wkly Rep.* 2023;72(37):1005–1009. https://doi.org/10.15585/mmwr.mm7237a2
7. Faherty EAG, Yuce D, Korban C, et al. Correlation of wastewater surveillance data with traditional influenza surveillance measures in Cook County, Illinois, October 2022–April 2023. *Sci Total Environ.* 2024;912:169551. https://doi.org/10.1016/j.scitotenv.2023.169551
8. Schoen ME, Bidwell AL, Wolfe MK, Boehm AB. United States influenza 2022–2023 season characteristics as inferred from wastewater solids, influenza hospitalization, and syndromic data. *Environ Sci Technol.* 2023;57(49):20542–20550. https://doi.org/10.1021/acs.est.3c07526
9. Toro L, de Valk H, Zanetti L, et al. Pathogen prioritisation for wastewater surveillance ahead of the Paris 2024 Olympic and Paralympic games, France. *Euro Surveill.* 2024;29(28): 2400231. https://doi.org/10.2807/1560-7917.ES.2024.29.28.2400231
10. Khalil AM, Martinez-Sobrido L, Mostafa A. Zoonosis and zooanthroponosis of emerging respiratory viruses. *Front Cell Infect Microbiol.* 2023;13:1232772. https://doi.org/10.3389/fcimb.2023.1232772
11. Centers for Disease Control and Prevention. How CDC is monitoring influenza data among people to better understand the current avian influenza A (H5N1) situation. 2024. Available at: https://www.cdc.gov/bird-flu/h5-monitoring/index.html. Accessed August 20, 2024.
12. Centers for Disease Control and Prevention. Influenza A virus wastewater data. 2024. Available at: https://www.cdc.gov/nwss/wastewater-surveillance/Flu-A-data.html. Accessed August 20, 2024.
13. Wolfe MK, Duong D, Shelden B, et al. Detection of hemagglutinin H5 influenza A virus sequence in municipal wastewater solids at wastewater treatment plants with increases in influenza A in spring, 2024. *Environ Sci Technol Lett.* 2024;11(6):526–532. https://doi.org/10.1021/acs.estlett.4c00331
14. Centers for Disease Control and Prevention. Calculating the wastewater viral activity level. Available at: https://www.cdc.gov/nwss/about-data.html#data-method. Accessed August 20, 2024.
15. Food and Drug Administration. Updates on highly pathogenic avian influenza (HPAI). 2024. Available at: https://www.fda.gov/food/alerts-advisories-safety-information/updates-highly-pathogenic-avian-influenza-hpai. Accessed June 30, 2024.
16. Nguyen T-Q, Hutter C, Markin A, et al. Emergence and interstate spread of highly pathogenic avian influenza A(H5N1) in dairy cattle. *bioRxiv.* 2024.2005.2001.591751. https://doi.org/10.1101/2024.05.01.591751
17. Lowry SA, Wolfe MK, Boehm AB. Respiratory virus concentrations in human excretions that contribute to wastewater: a systematic review and meta-analysis. *J Water Health.* 2023;21(6):831–848. https://doi.org/10.2166/wh.2023.057
18. Nelli RK, Harm TA, Siepker C, et al. Sialic acid receptor specificity in mammary gland of dairy cattle infected with highly pathogenic avian influenza A(H5N1) virus. *Emerg Infect Dis.* 2024;30(7): 1361–1373. https://doi.org/10.3201/eid3007.240689
19. Keenum I, Lin NJ, Logan-Jackson A, et al. Optimizing wastewater surveillance: the necessity of standardized reporting and proficiency for public health. *Am J Public Health.* 2024;114(9):859–863. https://doi.org/10.2105/AJPH.2024.307760
20. Louis S, Mark-Carew M, Biggerstaff M, et al. Wastewater surveillance for influenza A virus and H5 subtype concurrent with the highly pathogenic avian influenza A(H5N1) virus outbreak in cattle and poultry and associated human cases—United States, May 12–July 13, 2024. *MMWR Morb Mortal Wkly Rep.* 2024;73:804–809. https://www.cdc.gov/mmwr/volumes/73/wr/mm7337a1.htm?s_cid=mm7337a1_w
21. Lee AJ, Carson S, Reyne MI, et al. "One Health" genomic surveillance of avian and human influenza A viruses through environmental wastewater monitoring. *medRxiv.* 2023:2023.2008.2008.23293833. https://doi.org/10.1101/2023.08.08.23293833

Tracking Airborne Lead Exposures That Disrupt Children's Fronto-executive Functions and Inhibitory Systems

Lorenz S. Neuwirth, PhD

ABOUT THE AUTHOR

Lorenz S. Neuwirth, PhD, is a professor in the Department of Psychology at The State University of New York (SUNY) at Old Westbury, Old Westbury, NY. He is also a research professor in the SUNY Neuroscience Research Institute, Old Westbury.

Over the last 50 years, substantial efforts in the United States have been directed toward understanding the negative impacts of environmental lead exposures on children's brain development and their associated deficits in behavioral and intellectual functioning—specifically, fronto-executive and inhibitory dysfunctions.[1,2] Lead-poisoned children exhibit deficits in their attentional, emotional, learning, memory, and psychosocial functions that have maintained the public's interest in identifying and eliminating lead source exposures that continue to harm children in the United States. Despite these public health efforts to reduce lead source exposures (e.g., lead paint, leaded gasoline, lead emissions, and lead-based water and soil contaminants[3,4]), only recently has airborne lead exposures regained attention.[5]

NEW INSIGHTS ON AIRBORNE LEAD EXPOSURES

Gatzke-Kopp et al.[5] provided both compelling and concerning data warranting further study of airborne lead exposures that harm children to address this specific public health problem within the United States. Gatzke-Kopp et al.[5] replicated work from the Family Life Project and later examined the data from the Early Childhood Health Outcomes Cohort,[6] with an increased sample size covering a broader geographic, socioeconomic, and diverse population with all the attributes described therein (i.e., encompassing 188–237 counties across 36–41 states, from 69 ongoing pregnancy and pediatric cohort sites that evaluated children having at least three years of lead-exposure data). Their larger-scale study's findings showed a captivating epidemiological negative linear association between increased airborne lead exposures and decreased children's IQs and fronto-executive functions.[5] Moreover, their findings showed that the negative linear association specifically disrupted the brain's inhibitory systems,[5] which corroborated with preclinical reports.[7]

First, the implications of these findings suggest a general recommendation that could be useful in that children exposed to airborne lead could be tracked over time to evaluate reductions in their short- and long-term learning outcomes during their school-age years and increased economic costs when they become adults.[8] However, such data tracking would require a longitudinal study that might be costly. Second, perhaps creatively leveraging current real-time data systems already in place for lead as a primary pollutant within the ozone through an air quality index (AQI) by the Environmental Protection Agency (EPA; https://www.airnow.gov) and combining it with Reuters analytic approaches using the Centers for Disease Control and Prevention's (CDC's) nationwide analysis of children's blood lead levels (BLLs) obtained from neighborhood levels (https://www.reuters.com/investigates/graphics/lead-water/en) might serve to reduce costs and overcome the burdensome challenge of longitudinal participant tracking and dropout.

Although these two suggestions could increase our understanding of tracking lead-poisoned children in aggregates to localize efforts on where to intervene, they may come with the cost of limiting our ability for an individual child's tracking outcome. This trade-off at the sake of helping lead-poisoned children may still be useful, and if response efforts are deployed in a local area of concern, then outreach efforts may serve to capture these individual children through complementary or supplementary interventions. Notably, lead is a criteria air pollutant with a national monitoring network, yet it is not measured ubiquitously, and only a handful of states utilize the AQI. This limitation coupled with the inconsistent and highly variable BLL screening rates of children currently used can vary

AJPH December 2024, Vol. 114, No. 12

significantly by state and year,[9] making any approach seem promising at face value, but, in reality, it may fall short of a practical implementation method.

Furthermore, such a revamping of data-tracking systems, which have shown to be effective as the airborne lead exposure tracking, might improve state efforts to collect more accurate data on children's BLL screenings and increase more states' willingness to measure and track lead as an air pollutant through AQI. Notably, this revamping may present with a rather costly adaptation or deviation from current data-tracking methods regarding children's BLLs. Yet, improving upon the current tracking systems (i.e., the AQI and airborne lead measures) and standardizing them may reduce such costs and actually pay off in terms of the benefit–cost ratio.

LEAD EXPOSURE ECONOMIC LOSSES AND OPPORTUNITIES

What becomes apparent is that both the cost to adopt new and more accurate data tracking methods for childhood lead exposures and the accumulated long-term economic costs for supporting these same children through their education, their early intervention services, and other medical and mental health supports that persist into adulthood are clearly unsustainable.[3–5] Society will either pay more now for new data-tracking methods in an effort to proactively screen and reduce lead exposure from (re)occurring or pay a lot more later to reactively support these lead-poisoned children as they become adults. In addition, lead exposures serve as economic risk factors (e.g., adverse childhood experiences) that disproportionately affect marginalized, low-income, minority, and historically underserved populations[10,11] that often times live near industries, manufactories, or Superfund sites that have lower air quality.[12] Given the large push for artificial intelligence (AI) systems in big data science, there could be beneficial partnerships between the EPA, the CDC, and public health researchers to collaborate in meaningful ways to radically change the current practice of using children as inadequate biological detectors of lead exposures and poisoning.

Furthermore, what can be gleaned from the report by Gatzke-Kopp et al.[5] is that it would be prudent for the EPA to develop a timely data-tracking map of airborne lead exposures that could then be used by the CDC as a proxy to prompt local pediatricians in elevated exposure areas to conduct AQI-informed BLL screenings. This tripartite collaboration (i.e., EPA-CDC-pediatrician) through the data-tracking map could then be used to determine when and where an elevated airborne lead event occurred and inform the public of any "hot spots." This is important as the CDC consistently underreports children's' BLLs screenings, which, in turn, fall short of identifying where in the environment risks for lead source exposures are localized.[9]

Thus, a new approach to addressing airborne lead exposures has perhaps serendipitously re-emerged in the context of new data-tracking methodologies by Gatzke-Kopp et al.[5] to encourage and envision states to direct new resources toward developing a public-facing data-tracking mechanism for airborne lead exposures. This may not be an easy or practical financial cost, but conversations with state officials, public stakeholders, policymakers, and the federal government would all have to agree on the value of protecting the lives of children in the United States from ongoing lead exposures to resolve this problem. This is an unprecedented ask, but it may be the right time to begin the conversation and see where the dialogue directs states how to move forward in assessing and working toward realizing this goal. If federal and state grants could be designed to have calls directed toward developing such data-tracking systems and methodologies, this may alleviate some of the financial challenges associated with revamping the children's BLL screening data sets currently utilized. Thus, more grant money should be invested into research aimed at tracking airborne lead exposures and subsequently supporting public health response efforts to increase BLL screenings of all children, especially in areas with elevated airborne lead exposures.

A PARADIGM SHIFT FOR FUTURE LEAD-EXPOSURE RESEARCH

The childhood lead neurotoxicity field is undergoing a paradigm shift from the last 50 years that neurodevelopmental consequences of lead poisoning are treatable. This new perspective places greater responsibility on the federal and state government to inform the public on lead source exposures including airborne exposures. The last 50 years of study on children's cognitive and behavioral profiles with low-level lead exposures from birth to 6 years of age showed impairment, disruption, and deficits in the inhibitory and related fronto-executive systems that corroborate with the report by Gatzke-Kopp et al.[5]

In addition to airborne lead exposure data tracking and prompting more precise BLL screenings in children, complementary research may need to extend beyond the traditional work of targeting the glutamatergic learning and memory systems broadly linked to intellectual deficits caused by lead poisoning. Rather, a more intentional effort to better refine (pre)clinical approaches to understand the more nuanced GABAergic neural circuitry responsible for regulating both inhibition and disinhibition that is also linked to lead-induced deficits in intellectual, psycho-social-emotional, and behavioral outcomes. This becomes especially concerning as children age across the lifespan and their inhibition and disinhibition systems become more susceptible for later-life neurodevelopmental disorders mediated by the efficiency, or lack thereof, of the GABAergic system, and the current population is living much longer than previous generations. It is conceivable to consider that children and more senior populations are at elevated risk for lead-induced GABAergic problems. Thus, compounded economic costs may be incurred for both inhibitory problems observed in lead-poisoned children and later in their lives as adults.

Perhaps a parallel approach to addressing the risk of children being exposed to airborne lead in an environment from which they cannot relocate could be approached with a drug therapy that reduces the extent of harm lead has on the child's developing and maturing brain. An approach of this kind would also require substantial state and federal grants to stimulate the next decade of research from 2030 to 2040 to direct its effort toward more GABAergic inhibitory study as a proactive measure. Whether the federal and state governments decide to fund grants that stimulate early preclinical drug discovery for GABAergic treatments for lead poisoning or new big data tracking systems using AI between the EPA and CDC with talented public health researchers and pediatricians remains to be determined.

CONCLUSION

In the interim, public health researchers can decide to work voluntarily on developing an airborne lead–tracking system to help localize where reactive measures ought to occur in their states to map "hot spots" and using the CDC's available data sets to produce similar data that predict the negative association risks reported by Gatzke-Kopp et al.[5] Alternatively, preclinical researchers can work voluntarily to develop GABAergic drugs to address symptoms of lead poisoning. It is my opinion that if these proactive and reactive approaches were grant-funded and addressed simultaneously, society may avoid taking another 50 years to come to the conclusion that tracking airborne lead exposures could be used as a proxy for mapping areas in which children may be at risk for lead poisoning. Such an approach could serve to accurately track and provide early childhood drug treatment and public health interventions directed toward preserving children's fronto-executive and inhibitory systems while improving their quality of life. Taken together, my opinion to advocate such an approach may serve to concurrently reduce the unfortunate economic expenses and costs of more generations of children left lead-poisoned.[8] AJPH

CORRESPONDENCE

Correspondence should be sent to Lorenz S. Neuwirth, PhD, Professor, Psychology, SUNY Old Westbury, Department of Psychology, 223 Store Hill Rd, Old Westbury, NY 11568 (e-mail: neuwirthl@oldwestbury.edu). Reprints can be ordered at https://www.ajph.org by clicking the "Reprints" link.

PUBLICATION INFORMATION

Full Citation: Neuwirth LS. Tracking airborne lead exposures that disrupt children's fronto-executive functions and inhibitory systems. *Am J Public Health*. 2024;114(12):1313–1316.

Acceptance Date: September 4, 2024.

DOI: https://doi.org/10.2105/AJPH.2024.307866

ORCID iD:

Lorenz S. Neuwirth https://orcid.org/0000-0002-8194-522X

ACKNOWLEDGMENTS

This editorial was supported, in part, by a Faculty Development Grant awarded to L. S. Neuwirth.

CONFLICTS OF INTEREST

The author declares no potential or actual conflicts of interest from any funding or affiliation-related activities.

REFERENCES

1. White RF, Reuben AS. Environmental toxicities, including lead. In: Brown GG, King TZ, Haaland KY, Crosson B, eds. *APA Handbook of Neuropsychology, Vol. 1. Neurobehavioral Disorders and Conditions: Accepted Science and Open Questions*. Washington, DC: American Psychological Association; 2023:669–688. https://doi.org/10.1037/0000307-031
2. Neuwirth LS, Lopez OE, Schneider JS, Markowitz ME. Low-level lead exposure impairs fronto-executive functions: a call to update the *DSM-5* with lead poisoning as a neurodevelopmental disorder. *Psychol Neurosci*. 2020;13(3):299–325. https://doi.org/10.1037/pne0000225
3. Levin R, Schwartz J. A better cost:benefit analysis yields better results: the US Lead in Drinking Water Rule. *Environ Res*. 2023;229:115738. https://doi.org/10.1016/j.envres.2023.115738
4. Mielke HW, Egendorf SP. Getting the lead out: a career-long perspective on leaded gasoline, dust, soil, and proactive pediatric exposure prevention. *Med Res Arch*. 2023;11(5). https://doi.org/10.18103/mra.v11i5.3813
5. Gatzke-Kopp LM, Willoughby M, McArthur K, et al. Airborne lead exposure and childhood cognition: the Environmental Influences on Child Health Outcomes (ECHO) cohort (2003–2022). *Am J Public Health*. 2024;114(3):309–318. https://doi.org/10.2105/AJPH.2023.307519
6. Knapp EA, Kress AM, Parker CB, et al. The Environmental Influences on Child Health Outcomes (ECHO)-wide cohort. *Am J Epidemiol*. 2023;192(8):1249–1263. https://doi.org/10.1093/aje/kwad071
7. Neuwirth LS. *The Characterization of Pb2+ Toxicity in Rat Neural Development: An Assessment of Pb2+ Effects on the GABA Shift in Neural Networks and Implications for Learning and Memory Disruption*. Dissertation. CUNY Graduate Center; April 2014. Available at: https://academicworks.cuny.edu/gc_etds/82. Accessed September 17, 2024.
8. McFarland MJ, Hauer ME, Reuben A. Half of US population exposed to adverse lead levels in early

childhood. *Proc Natl Acad Sci U S A.* 2022;119(11): e2118631119. https://doi.org/10.1073/pnas.2118631119

9. Neuwirth LS. Resurgent lead poisoning and renewed public attention towards environmental social justice issues: a review of current efforts and call to revitalize primary and secondary lead poisoning prevention for pregnant women, lactating mothers, and children within the US. *Int J Occup Environ Health.* 2018;24(3-4):86–100. https://doi.org/10.1080/10773525.2018.1507291
10. Dickerson AS, Frndak S, DeSantiago M, Mohan A, Smith GS. Environmental exposure disparities and neurodevelopmental risk: a review. *Curr Environ Health Rep.* 2023;10(2):73–83. https://doi.org/10.1007/s40572-023-00396-6
11. Neuwirth LS, Whigham K. "Only time will tell": the underexplored impacts of lead poisoning and COVID-19 on pre-existing ACES in New York. *Youth.* 2023;3(4):1212–1224. https://doi.org/10.3390/youth3040077
12. Kerr GH, van Donkelaar A, Martin RV, et al. Increasing racial and ethnic disparities in ambient air pollution—attributable morbidity and mortality in the United States. *Environ Health Perspect.* 2024;132(3):37002. https://doi.org/10.1289/EHP11900

Breaking Down Silos Within a Multihospital System: Lessons From the California Department of State Hospitals' Response to the COVID-19 Pandemic

Maria I. Ventura, PhD, Robert Schaufenbil, Thanhtuyen Do, MD, Juan Carlos Arguello, DO, Jane Siegel, MD, and Katherine Warburton, DO

The California Department of State Hospitals and Department of Public Health collaborated to develop infection control programs in five inpatient psychiatric hospitals in response to COVID-19. In the retrospective observational study described here, conducted from March 2020 through February 2023, we calculated seven-day rolling averages of COVID-19 cases overlaid with key interventions, communication strategies, and policies implemented to break down silos for a consistent and coordinated response. Our findings may inform others regarding effective strategies and partnerships with public health experts during future outbreaks. (*Am J Public Health*. 2024;114(12):1317–1321. https://doi.org/10.2105/AJPH.2024.307846)

AJPH December 2024, Vol. 114, No. 12

Identifying effective interventions and key implementation strategies is critical for any health care system to respond to a public health emergency.

INTERVENTION AND IMPLEMENTATION

The COVID-19 pandemic necessitated that health care systems strike a balance between caring for sick patients and implementing infection control measures to limit transmission of severe acute respiratory syndrome coronavirus 2 (SARS-CoV-2). Individuals 50 years and older in long-term care facilities were among the most vulnerable and experienced the greatest impact of any group during the early stages of the pandemic.[1] As the pandemic persisted, other congregate settings such as long-term psychiatric inpatient hospitals and correctional facilities also faced unique challenges responding to outbreaks.[2,3] It has been shown that individuals with neuropsychiatric disorders exhibit poor adherence to infection control measures, including maintaining adequate spatial distancing and wearing protective face coverings.[4] The increased risk of morbidity and mortality associated with COVID-19 among patients with neuropsychiatric disorders is magnified by the increased rates of underlying health comorbidities.[5,6]

The California Department of State Hospitals (DSH), composed of five geographically separated and independently operated hospitals with headquarters in Sacramento, serves the largest number of forensic psychiatric inpatients in any US state with a bed capacity of 6082 and a total workforce of more than 10 000 (Table 1). Fifty-four percent of our patients have one or more medical risk factors (e.g., advanced age, underlying health conditions) that elevate their risk of severe outcomes if they develop COVID-19.[7] Furthermore, individuals are housed in shared sleeping quarters with shared bathrooms and living spaces, making it difficult to prevent transmission of SARS-CoV-2.

PLACE, TIME, AND PERSONS

We conducted a retrospective observational study of COVID-19 cases in California from March 8, 2020, through February 28, 2023. DSH collaborated

TABLE 1— Comparison of the Characteristics of Five Psychiatric State Hospitals: California, 2020–2023

	COVID-19 Region					
Characteristic	Bay Area (Facility 1)	San Joaquin Valley (Facility 2)	Southern California (Facility 3)	Bay Area (Facility 4)	Southern California (Facility 5)	Total
Total beds available, no.	1 108	1 380	935	1 203	1 456	6 082
No. of skilled nursing facility beds	0	0	96	29	0	125
Unique patients served (Mar 8, 2020–Feb 28, 2023), no.	3 908	1 684	3 219	3 310	3 093	15 214
Male patients, %	100	100	85	77	71	86
Length of stay, d, mean ± SD	313 ± 376	2 323 ± 2 506	265 ± 596	577 ± 1367	691 ± 1 429	540 ± 1 140
Patient age, y, mean ± SD	43 ± 12.5	57 ± 11.9	43 ± 14.5	49.5 ± 15.2	48.5 ± 14.0	41.7 ± 13.1
Patients with one or more COVID risk factors, no. (%[a])	2 039 (52)	1 351 (80)	1 409 (44)	1 829 (55)	1 549 (50)	8 177 (54)
Cumulative patient positive cases (Mar 8, 2020–Feb 28, 2023), no.	725	1 343	965	853	1 728	5 614
Cumulative staff positive cases (Mar 8, 2020–Feb 28, 2023), no.	1 675	2 203	1 949	1 927	2 648	10 402
Average no. of staff members working in each facility[b]	1 829	2 060	1 906	2 165	2 653	10 613

Note. Two of the five hospitals have skilled nursing facility units, and two house male patients only. Lengths of stay and the average age of patients vary by hospital. The percentage of patients with one or more COVID-19 risk factors ranged from 44% to 80%.
[a]No. of patients with one or more COVID risk factors/no. of patients served during study time frame.
[b]This information (as of April 2024) is an estimate and does not capture staffing throughout the pandemic, nor does it include contractors or temporary staff.

with the California Department of Public Health (CDPH) in developing COVID-19-specific guidance for infection prevention and control, testing, and vaccination and therapeutic programs throughout various waves of the pandemic. Medical epidemiologists and infection preventionists from the CDPH Healthcare-Associated Infections Program provided regular consultations through onsite infection control assessments, virtual meetings, and reviews of written recommendations for limiting SARS-CoV-2 transmission.

PURPOSE

Our goal is to share lessons learned from our collaboration with CDPH to develop programs mitigating transmission and adverse effects of COVID-19. These programs might serve as a model for inpatient psychiatric facilities with vulnerable populations to optimize care in future public health emergencies.

EVALUATION AND ADVERSE EFFECTS

Throughout various waves of the COVID-19 pandemic, our multihospital system had to execute a coordinated response to continue caring for patients while also addressing the public health needs of our system.

Infection Control and Communication

Our descriptive analysis included a timeline of COVID-19 interventions, communication strategies, and policies implemented overlaid on a seven-day rolling average of patient and staff COVID-19 cases across five DSH facilities (Figure 1). DSH patient case rates (daily patient positives/total patients served × 1000) were compared with case rates from another statewide inpatient psychiatric hospital system that also implemented antigen testing for patients and staff members during the pandemic.[8]

Frequent communication with hospital staff was imperative for efficient hospital operations, especially during the early stages of the pandemic when rapid action was needed to implement a robust infection control response. On March 2, 2020, California's governor issued a proclamation of a state of emergency that prompted DSH to activate six separate hospital incident command systems (one from each hospital and one at headquarters) on March 8. A unified hospital command group was convened on March 20 and met each day for one hour to coordinate a DSH response to the rapidly changing situation.

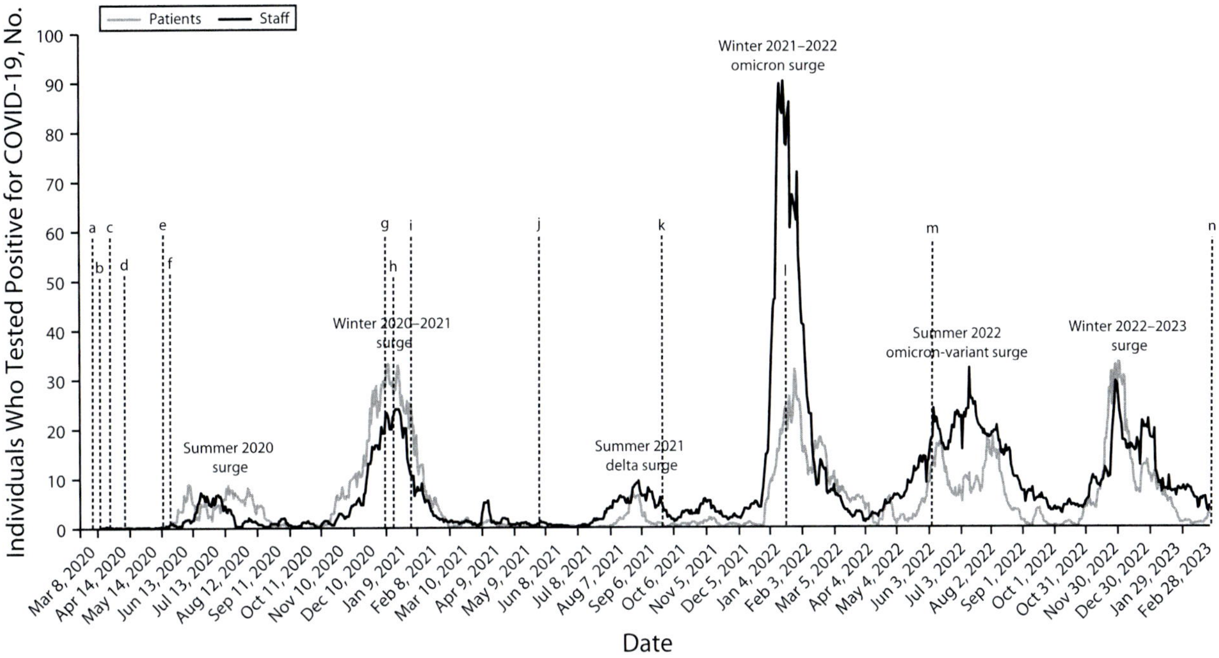

FIGURE 1— Seven-Day Rolling Average of Patient and Staff COVID-19 Cases in the Department of State Hospitals Overlaid With Key COVID-19 Interventions and Policies Implemented Between March 8, 2020, and the End of the California State of Emergency on February 28, 2023

Note. PCR = polymerase chain reaction.
a. Hospital Incident Command System activated during the week of March 8, 2020.
b. Hospital visitation halted March 12, 2020.
c. Unified Hospital Command Group convened on March 20, 2020.
d. Employee support line activated, and universal masks rolled out to staff and patients on March 26, 2020.
e. Healthcare-Associated Infections Program partnership commenced on May 15, 2020.
f. Admission observation units activated on May 22, 2020.
g. Daily rapid antigen testing for staff commenced on December 16, 2020.
h. Vaccination campaign began for staff on December 26, 2020.
i. Vaccination campaign began for patients on January 7, 2021.
j. PCR testing switched to the Color Laboratory Network on May 1, 2021.
k. Booster vaccinations for immunocompromised patients initiated on September 2, 2021.
l. Therapeutics initiated at all five state hospitals on January 19, 2022.
m. Cepheid analyzers for rapid PCR testing activated on-site at all five state hospitals on June 1, 2022.
n. End of California state of emergency and daily rapid antigen testing and switch to symptom-based testing on February 28, 2023.

Numerous protocols were developed with the guidance of CDPH Healthcare-Associated Infections Program public health experts, including use of personal protective equipment, cohort-based admission procedures, and quarantine, isolation, and testing strategies. DSH temporarily suspended admissions and discharges for all patient commitment types allowable under state law from March 16 through May 21, 2020, to implement infection control mitigation practices. On May 22, DSH resumed admissions by placing patient cohorts in converted admission observation units for 14 days, allowing for symptom monitoring and serial testing for the duration of the presumed incubation of the circulating strain.

The unified hospital command group communicated all information through multiple channels to ensure dissemination, including virtual townhalls and a pandemic-specific intranet site that provided COVID-19 fact sheets, links to financial assistance programs and local county public health departments, and stress reduction and emotional support resources (e.g., grief and loss, guided meditation). Furthermore, an employee support line was activated on March 26, 2020, and was available around the clock to answer questions and provide emotional support and connections to self-care or child-care services. Nearly 2000 contacts were made through the employee support line.

Testing

DSH had minimal access to COVID-19 testing until October 2020, when CDPH established a centralized laboratory to manage large volumes of polymerase chain reaction (PCR) tests. DSH began conducting all PCR testing for staff and patients through this centralized laboratory with turnaround times averaging two to three days. In May 2021, CDPH (and thus DSH) transitioned to the Color Laboratory Network, resulting in faster turnaround times averaging 24 to 34 hours. In June 2022, DSH acquired five GeneXpert Xpress Cepheid Analyzers for each facility to detect the SARS-CoV-2 virus via rapid PCR.[9] Here we present seven-day rolling average of positive cases among staff and patients from March 15, 2020, to the end of the state of emergency proclamation on February 28, 2023 (Figure 1). Each facility and its resident population had unique characteristics (e.g., geographic location, age of the patient population) that likely contributed to the overall number of COVID-19 cases during the pandemic (Table 1).

As more knowledge was gained about the utility of rapid antigen testing in identifying infectious individuals more rapidly than with PCR testing,[10,11] DSH consulted with the CDPH testing task force and the Healthcare-Associated Infections Program to implement a daily rapid antigen testing program for all direct-care hospital staff. This program, initiated on December 16, 2020, allowed for early identification of infected staff members before their start of shift. By the end of the California state of emergency proclamation, 2 668 233 antigen tests had been administered to DSH staff.[12] Before the implementation of rapid testing, the DSH case rate was 2.17 (per 1000 patients). A month after we began universal antigen testing for staff, our patient case rate decreased nearly 66% to 0.74. These findings are comparable to New York State–operated psychiatric hospitals that reported a 60% decrease in patient case rates (from 2.02 to 0.81) after initiation of voluntary antigen testing.[8]

Vaccines

After the Pfizer BioNTech (BNT162b2) and Moderna (mRNA-1273) vaccines were granted emergency use authorizations, DSH established a robust vaccine campaign on December 26, 2020, for staff and January 7, 2021, for patients. No serious vaccine side effects or complications were observed. By the end of the California state of emergency proclamation, DSH had achieved 82% primary series vaccination rates among staff and 69% among patients, as compared with a 72.8% vaccination rate with the primary series among the population of California.[13]

Therapeutics

On January 19, 2022, DSH received Food and Drug Administration–authorized monoclonal antibodies from CDPH to provide long-acting preexposure prophylaxis for immunocompromised patients. Between February 14 and February 28, our hospitals began receiving therapeutic antiviral agents. Therapeutic treatments were highly efficacious in treating mild to moderate COVID-19 infections; less than 0.03% of our patients required acute intensive care treatment, and those who were transferred out all had complicating comorbidities.

SUSTAINABILITY

Each infection control intervention implemented within our system was imperfect, much like the Swiss cheese defense described by Reason.[14] However, layered together, these interventions gave us a robust defense against COVID-19.[15] The prompt activation of the unified hospital command group broke down silos within DSH, allowing us to implement consistent infection control practices across hospitals and respond to the pandemic in a coordinated fashion. The comprehensive intranet site regularly offered employees updates and resources, and the employee support line and virtual town halls provided a steady bidirectional stream of communication between front-line employees and hospital leaders. Daily rapid antigen testing for all direct-care staff was instrumental in reducing the number of infectious individuals entering our high-risk facilities and exposing vulnerable patients, thereby potentially reducing outbreaks and preventing morbidity and mortality.

For example, during summer 2020 and winter 2020–2021, before the initiation of universal testing of patients and staff, patient positivity rates often exceeded staff positivity rates. However, through subsequent surges, patient positivity rates remained lower than overall staff rates. More than 60% of individuals who tested positive via rapid antigen tests were asymptomatic and would have otherwise attended work while infectious. We believe that antigen testing was a robust defense against COVID-19 entering and spreading throughout our vulnerable facilities, comparable to what was observed in New York State psychiatric hospitals that conducted widespread antigen testing for patients and staff members.[8] Our partnership with local and state public health departments allowed us to implement infection control measures that mitigated the risk of transmission and severe outcomes in our system despite patient vulnerabilities.

PUBLIC HEALTH SIGNIFICANCE

The impact of the COVID-19 pandemic on congregate health care facilities housing vulnerable patients had the potential to become a devastating mass causality event. Although our response was not perfect, our leadership team embraced changes to infection control practices in full partnership with public health experts. Broad and sustained testing and vaccination efforts are costly and time sensitive, and they may garner skepticism. However, we believe that these efforts were correlated with reductions in outbreak severity in our system and thus worth the investment. Effective communication strategies broke down silos between our sites and allowed a systematized approach to COVID-19. Our findings can guide future responses to public health emergencies in other high transmission risk settings such as schools or hospital systems. AJPH

ABOUT THE AUTHORS

At the time of the study, the authors were with the California Department of State Hospitals and the California Department of Public Health, Sacramento.

CORRESPONDENCE

Correspondence should be sent to Maria I. Ventura, PhD, 1215 O St, Sacramento, CA 95814 (e-mail: maria.ventura@dsh.ca.gov). Reprints can be ordered at https://www.ajph.org by clicking the "Reprints" link.

PUBLICATION INFORMATION

Full Citation: Ventura MI, Schaufenbil R, Do T, Arguello JC, Siegel J, Warburton K. Breaking down silos within a multihospital system: lessons from the California Department of State Hospitals' response to the COVID-19 pandemic. *Am J Public Health*. 2024;114(12):1317–1321.

Acceptance Date: August 9, 2024.

DOI: https://doi.org/10.2105/AJPH.2024.307846

CONTRIBUTORS

M. I. Ventura contributed to the design and to analysis and interpretation of the data and drafted and revised content. R. Schaufenbil and T. Do contributed to drafting and revising content. J. C. Arguello, J. Siegel, and K. Warburton contributed to the conception and design of the study and reviewed content.

ACKNOWLEDGMENTS

We express our gratitude for our partnership with California Department of Public Health groups including the Healthcare-Associated Infections Program and the testing, vaccine, and therapeutics task forces.

Note. The findings and conclusions in this article are those of the authors and do not necessarily represent the views or opinions of the California Department of State Hospitals or the California Health and Human Services Agency.

CONFLICTS OF INTEREST

The authors have no conflicts of interest to report.

HUMAN PARTICIPANT PROTECTION

This research was approved by the California Health and Human Services Committee for the Protection of Human Subjects. A waiver of informed consent was granted for this protocol because only preexisting hospital surveillance data were used.

REFERENCES

1. Callaghan AW, Chard AN, Arnold P, et al. Screening for SARS-CoV-2 infection within a psychiatric hospital and considerations for limiting transmission within residential psychiatric facilities. *MMWR Morb Mortal Wkly Rep*. 2020;69(26):825–829. https://doi.org/10.15585/mmwr.mm6926a4
2. Dykgraaf SH, Matenge S, Desborough J, et al. Protecting nursing homes and long-term care facilities from COVID-19: a rapid review of international evidence. *J Am Med Dir Assoc*. 2021;22:1969–1988.
3. Frazer K, Mitchell L, Stokes D, Lacey E, Crowley E, Kelleher CC. A rapid systematic review of measures to protect older people in long-term care facilities from COVID-19. *BMJ Open*. 2021;11(10):e047012. https://doi.org/10.1136/bmjopen-2020-047012
4. Williams R, Tweed J, Rebolledo L, Khalid O, Agyeman J, Pinto da Costa M. Patient adherence with infection control measures on a novel 'COVID-19 triage' psychiatric in-patient ward. *BJPsych Open*. 2021;7(4):e131. https://doi.org/10.1192/bjo.2021.968
5. Toubasi AA, AbuAnzeh RB, Tawileh HB, Aldebei RH, Alryalat SAS. A meta-analysis: the mortality and severity of COVID-19 among patients with mental disorders. *Psychiatry Res*. 2021;299:113856. https://doi.org/10.1016/j.psychres.2021.113856
6. Das-Munshi J. Severe mental illness, race/ethnicity, multimorbidity and mortality following COVID-19 infection: nationally representative cohort study. *Br J Psychiatry*. 2023;223(5):518–525. https://doi.org/10.1192/bjp.2023.112
7. Centers for Disease Control and Prevention. Factors that affect your risk of getting very sick from COVID-19. Available at: https://archive.cdc.gov/#/details?q=https://www.cdc.gov/coronavirus/2019-ncov/your-health/risks-getting-very-sick.html&start=0&rows=10&url=https://www.cdc.gov/coronavirus/2019-ncov/your-health/risks-getting-very-sick.html. Accessed June 20, 2024.
8. Smith TE, Rodgers IT, Silverman DJ, et al. COVID-19 case rates after surveillance and vaccinations in a statewide psychiatric hospital system. *Am J Public Health*. 2021;111(10):1780–1783. https://doi.org/10.2105/AJPH.2021.306444
9. Lee J, Song J. Diagnostic accuracy of the Cepheid Xpert Xpress and the Abbott ID NOW assay for rapid detection of SARS-CoV-2: a systemic review and meta-analysis. *J Med Virol*. 2021;93(7):4523–4531. https://doi.org/10.1002/jmv.26994
10. Chin ET, Huynh BQ, Chapman LAC, Murrill M, Basu S, Lo NC. Frequency of routine testing for coronavirus disease 2019 (COVID-19) in high-risk healthcare environments to reduce outbreaks. *Clin Infect Dis*. 2021;73(9):e3127–e3129. https://doi.org/10.1093/cid/ciaa1383
11. Fouzas S. SARS-CoV-2 rapid antigen detection tests. *Lancet Infect Dis*. 2021;21(8):1068–1069. https://doi.org/10.1016/S1473-3099(21)00206-1
12. Ventura MI, Delgado D, Velasquez S, et al. Large-scale implementation of a daily rapid antigen testing program in California for detecting SARS-CoV-2. *Am J Public Health*. 2022;112(3):467–471. https://doi.org/10.2105/AJPH.2021.306588
13. California Department of Public Health. COVID-19 home page. Available at: https://covid19.ca.gov. Accessed June 20, 2024.
14. Reason J. Human error: models and management. *BMJ*. 2000;320(7237):768–770. https://doi.org/10.1136/bmj.320.7237.768
15. McKay IM. The Swiss cheese respiratory virus defense. Available at: https://figshare.com/articles/figure/The_Swiss_Cheese_Respiratory_Virus_Defence/13082618?file=25233461. Accessed June 20, 2024.

Media Communications Must Promote Healthy Hydration Policies and Environments That Encourage Water Consumption to Reduce Sugary Beverage Health Risks

Vivica I. Kraak, RDN, PhD, MS, and Nicole L. Furr, MS

ABOUT THE AUTHORS

Vivica I. Kraak and Nicole L. Furr are with the Department of Human Nutrition, Foods, and Exercise, Virginia Polytechnic Institute and State University (Virginia Tech), Blacksburg.

See also State Laws Targeting Marginalized Groups, pp. 1326–1364.

"When the Coca-Cola Company wants to change behavior, it does not hire professional counselors; it beams us evocative images. When we want to reduce smoking or reverse a national epidemic of obesity, so should we."

—*Thomas Farley, MD, MPH*[1]

Robust evidence shows that the widespread marketing of branded sugary beverages has contributed to undernutrition, obesity, and chronic noncommunicable diseases for populations, and to plastic pollution that accelerates climate change.[2] Persuasive appeals are used in messages, taglines, and slogans for media campaigns to change people's hearts, minds, and behaviors.[3,4] Persuasive appeals could be used within a broader social change movement to socially normalize policies and environments that encourage healthy eating and safe drinking water and that discourage sugary beverages.[3,4]

In this issue of *AJPH*, Grummon et al. (p. 1354) implemented an online randomized controlled trial to assess the effectiveness of countermarketing versus health education messages on adults' perceived weight stigma and intention to consume sugary drinks in the United States. This study tested countermarketing messages that reduced adults' intention to consume sugary beverages without reinforcing weight stigma compared with health education messages. The study adds to growing evidence that countermarketing messages may discourage short-term sugary beverage buying and consumption.

However, most American children, adolescents, and adults are exposed daily to a cacophony of conflicting messages online and in retail settings about which beverages to drink for optimal healthy hydration.[3,4] Many Americans experience water insecurity in US cities and rural communities,[5] which may lead them to buy and consume plastic bottled water or soda, a behavior exacerbated by climate change.

The Coca-Cola Company, PepsiCo, Inc., and Keurig Dr. Pepper market hundreds of brands and thousands of beverage products to people, including sugary and artificially sweetened carbonated sodas, fruit drinks, flavored dairy and plant-based milks, flavored sparkling and carbonated water, sweetened coffees and teas, sports and energy drinks, and functional beverages.[3,6] The global, ready-to-drink, nonalcoholic beverage market is valued at US $1.8 trillion in 2024 and may reach US $3.8 trillion by 2034.[6]

Public health luminaries have emphasized the power of using mass media communications to achieve population health goals. Farley[1] discussed the Internet fostering a digital communications revolution where social media and smartphones have created new opportunities to reach people anywhere, anytime. Green and Kreuter[7] described mass media campaigns used in synergistic, multicomponent tobacco control efforts that helped to denormalize the tobacco industry's marketing practices, raise public awareness, and mobilize community support for governments to tax tobacco products, and enact laws for smoke-free workplaces, restaurants, and outdoor public settings.[7]

Chapman[8] offered advice to early career public health advocates to design effective media advocacy

AJPH December 2024, Vol. 114, No. 12

campaigns, including (1) be clear and concrete about what you want to change or support; (2) study how social media works, how you can use it, and use it a lot; (3) use killer facts, and identify values that make these facts compelling; (4) understand your opponents' vulnerability and strategically reframe values positively; and (5) be patient, because effective advocacy takes time.[8]

A study that evaluated 280 US media campaigns (1886–2021) found that two thirds were dominated by beverage firms' corporate advertising and marketing for branded sugary beverages that used positive emotional appeals (65.8%; n = 184 campaigns).[3,4] Coca-Cola and PepsiCo, Inc. have used attractive graphic images, slogans, and taglines in marketing communications for more than a century to build intergenerational brand loyalty for sugary beverages that are deeply embedded in American culture.[3,4] Countermarketing and media advocacy campaigns (3.6%; n = 10 campaigns)[3] used rational appeals as well as positive and negative emotional appeals, and health education campaigns used negative emotional appeals (48%) to highlight sugary beverage harms. Public policy campaigns combined positive emotional and rational appeals to motivate actions to support or oppose sugary beverage tax legislation.[3,4]

US public health practitioners and community activists must aspire to a more ambitious vision that uses positive persuasive media communications to urge decisionmakers to support healthy hydration policies and environments that ensure safe free potable water as the healthy default beverage. Figure 1 shows six research priorities to advance evidence about persuasive message framing to develop strategic communications to reduce sugary beverage health risks for Americans.[3]

The challenges ahead are extensive. By 2024, the United States had made no measurable progress to achieve the Healthy People 2030 objective to reduce added sugars consumed by individuals aged two and older from 13.5% to 11.5%, which translates to six to 12 teaspoons of added sugars consumed daily.[9] Healthy hydration and water security were not included in the 2022 National Strategy to improve nutrition security for Americans. Between 2011 and 2024, the federal government failed to enact a national sugary beverage excise tax despite the SWEET Act bill introduced into several Congressional sessions.

Industry-funded efforts at the state level to preempt sugary beverage taxes have prevented new local sugary beverage legislation since 2018, which raises the urgency to effectively mobilize diverse citizen coalitions to reduce sugary beverage health risks.[10,11] The United States ranks below 35 countries that promoted policy coherence by enacting national sugary beverage tax legislation and developing strong heathy hydration recommendations that encourage water and discourage sugary beverages.[12]

Chapman[8] advised that we must be clear about what to change and use killer facts that could be used in positive persuasive communications delivered through integrated print, broadcast, and digital media to educate, inform, and advocate for three priority actions. First, public health activists must urge the US Department of Agriculture (USDA) and Health and Human Services to establish healthy hydration recommendations across the lifespan in the Dietary Guidelines for Americans 2025–2030, and the USDA should update the MyPlate graphic to show water as the healthy default beverage and discourage sugary beverages.[12] Second, public health activists should encourage government agencies to use the updated dietary guidelines to ensure policy coherence for healthy hydration in programs, settings, and sectors. Third, public health activist coalitions should urge legislators to pass national sugary beverage tax legislation in the 119th US Congress (2025–2027).

Persuasive communications, media advocacy, and public policy campaigns should highlight these killer facts: New York City's mayor signed the SWEET Truth Act into law in 2023 that, starting in September 2024, required chain restaurants to display warning icons for fountain beverages and other items that exceed the maximum daily target for added sugars (50 g or 12 teaspoons)[13]; and sugary beverage tax legislation evaluations have shown substantially reduced purchases in five US cities[14] and lowered youth obesity risk.[15]

Global public health activists are bundling health, environmental, and equity issues and climate justice into multicultural and multilingual digital media advocacy and policy campaigns to counter corporate advertising and public relations campaigns. In July 2024, the Kick Big Soda Out of Sport campaign[16] challenged Coca-Cola's It's Magic When the World Comes Together campaign[17] launched for the Olympic and Paralympic Games in Paris. By September 2024, Kick Big Soda Out mobilized over 255 600 citizens to sign and share an online petition, and 93 partner organizations urged the International Olympic Committee to end its long-term sponsorship of international sports events and athletes with Coca-Cola, which harms the health of

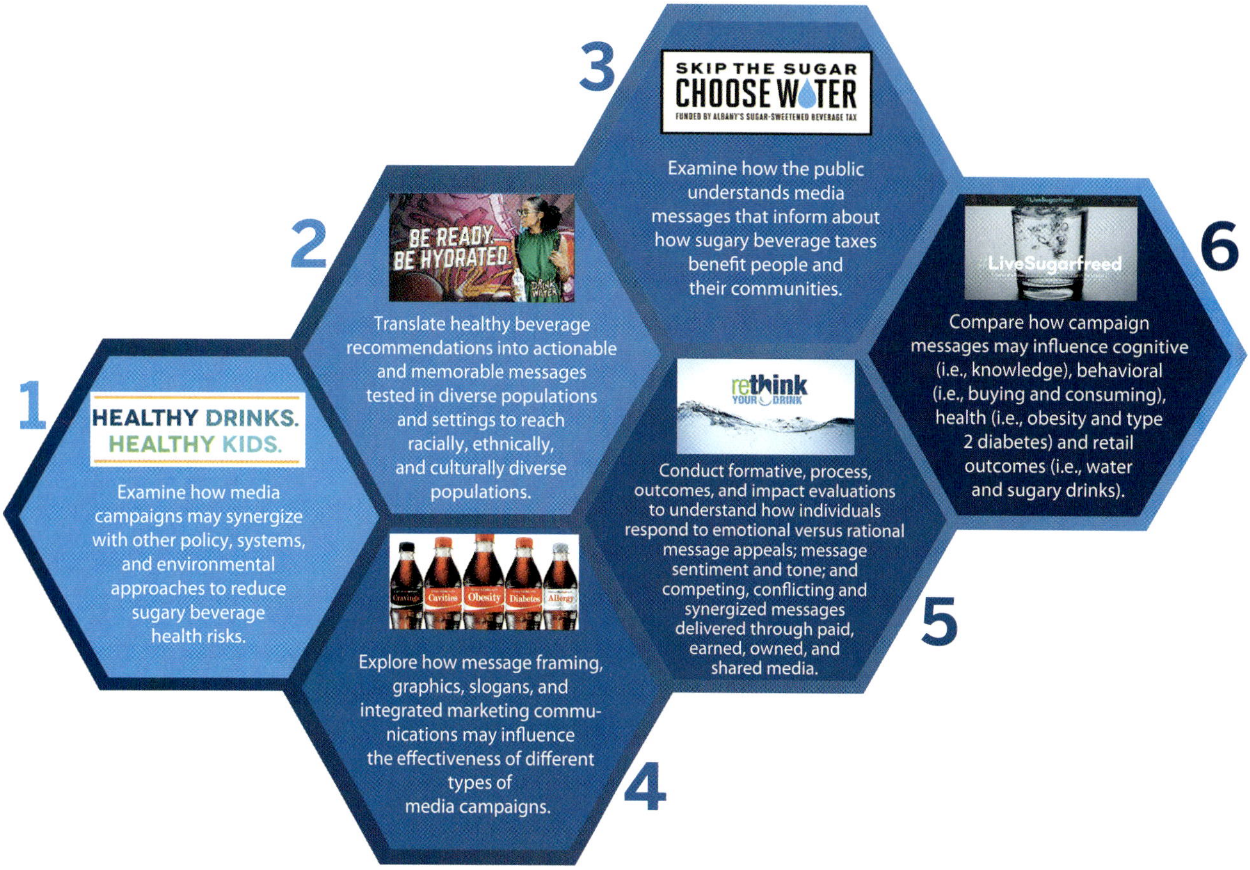

FIGURE 1— Research Priorities for Generating Evidence to Develop Strategic Media Communications to Reduce Sugary Beverage Health Risks

Note. The trademarked images used in this figure are intended for educational purposes only. Their use is allowed for non-commercial purposes through the US Copyright Office's Fair Use Law (https://www.copyright.gov/fair-use/more-info.html) that protects free speech over trademark infringement.
Source. Kraak et al.[3] The figure was reprinted with permission from the authors under a Creative Commons CC BY license.

people and damages the environment and planet.[16]

US policymakers, public health practitioners, private foundations, and scholar and youth activists have enormous but unrealized opportunities to unite efforts in coalitions and use digital media strategically to deliver persuasive communications that will support a social change movement that will urge healthy hydration policies and environments to provide safe, accessible drinking water and reduce sugary beverage health risks for Americans. AJPH

CORRESPONDENCE

Correspondence should be sent to Vivica I. Kraak, RDN, PhD, MS, Department of Human Nutrition, Foods, and Exercise, 257 Wallace Hall, 295 West Campus Dr, Virginia Polytechnic Institute and State University (Virginia Tech), Blacksburg, VA 24061 (e-mail: vivica51@vt.edu). Reprints can be ordered at https://www.ajph.org by clicking the "Reprints" link.

PUBLICATION INFORMATION

Full Citation: Kraak VI, Furr NL. Media communications must promote healthy hydration policies and environments that encourage water consumption to reduce sugary beverage health risks. *Am J Public Health*. 2024;114(12):1322–1325.

Acceptance Date: September 19, 2024.

DOI: https://doi.org/10.2105/AJPH.2024.307880

ORCID iDs:

Vivica I. Kraak https://orcid.org/0000-0002-9303-5530

Nicole L. Furr https://orcid.org/0000-0002-3110-3219

CONTRIBUTORS

V. I. Kraak conceptualized, researched, drafted, and revised the editorial. N. L. Furr reviewed and revised the editorial. Both authors approved the final submission.

ACKNOWLEDGMENTS

We thank Juan Quirarte for designing the figure published by *Obesity Reviews* in an open access article distributed under the terms of the Creative Commons CC BY license.

CONFLICTS OF INTEREST

The authors report no potential or actual conflicts of interest from funding or affiliation-related activities pertaining to this editorial.

REFERENCES

1. Farley TA. Mass diseases, mass exposures, and mass media. *JAMA Intern Med.* 2015;175(11): 1743–1744. https://doi.org/10.1001/jamainternmed.2015.5079
2. Malik VS, Hu FB. The role of sugar-sweetened beverages in the global epidemics of obesity and chronic diseases. *Nat Rev Endocrinol.* 2022;18(4): 205–218. https://doi.org/10.1038/s41574-021-00627-6
3. Kraak VI, Consavage Stanley K, Harrigan PB, Zhou M. How have media campaigns been used to promote and discourage healthy and unhealthy beverages in the United States? A systematic scoping review to inform future research to reduce sugary beverage health risks to Americans. *Obes Rev.* 2022;23(5):e13425. https://doi.org/10.1111/obr.13425
4. Kraak VI, Holz A, Woods CL, Whitlow AR, Leary N. A content analysis of persuasive appeals used in media campaigns to encourage and discourage sugary beverages and water in the United States. *Int J Environ Res Public Health.* 2023;20(14):6359. https://doi.org/10.3390/ijerph20146359
5. Meehan K, Jurjevich JR, Chun NMJW, Sherrill J. Geographies of insecure water access and the housing-water nexus in US cities. *Proc Natl Acad Sci USA.* 2020;117(46):28700–28707. https://doi.org/10.1073/pnas.2007361117
6. Global Newswire. Non-alcoholic beverage market projected to double by 2034, reaching a value of USD 3.8 trillion. August 21, 2024. Available at: https://www.globenewswire.com/news-release/2024/08/21/2933620/0/en/Non-Alcoholic-Beverage-Market-Projected-to-Double-by-2034-Reaching-a-Value-of-USD-3-8-Trillion.html. Accessed September 30, 2024.
7. Green LW, Kreuter MW. Evidence hierarchies versus synergistic interventions. *Am J Public Health.* 2010;100(10):1824–1825. https://doi.org/10.2105/AJPH.2010.197798
8. Chapman S. Reflections on a 38-year career in public health advocacy: 10 pieces of advice to early career researchers and advocates. *Public Health Res Pract.* 2015;25(2):e2521514. https://doi.org/10.17061/phrp2521514
9. Dept of Health and Human Services. Healthy People 2030. Reduce consumption of added sugars by people aged 2 years and over—NWS-10. Available at: https://health.gov/healthypeople/objectives-and-data/browse-objectives/nutrition-and-healthy-eating/reduce-consumption-added-sugars-people-aged-2-years-and-over-nws-10. Accessed August 24, 2024.
10. Falbe J, Adler SS, Roberto CA. Sugar-sweetened beverage tax preemption and the urgency of unified mobilization. *Am J Public Health.* 2021;111(4): 546–548. https://doi.org/10.2105/AJPH.2021.306163
11. Garibay KK, Burke NJ, Ramírez AS, Payán DD. Examining the role and strategies of advocacy coalitions in California's statewide sugar-sweetened beverage tax debate (2001–2018). *Am J Health Promot.* 2024;38(1):101–111. https://doi.org/10.1177/08901171231201007
12. Leary N, Parker MK, Rincón Gallardo Patiño S, Kraak VI. An evaluation of healthy hydration recommendations for 93 countries with sugary beverage tax legislation globally, 2000–2023. *Nutrients.* 2024;16(14):2264. https://doi.org/10.3390/nu16142264
13. Center for Science in the Public Interest. NYC Mayor Eric Adams signs Sweet Truth Act [press release]. November 17, 2023. Available at: https://www.cspinet.org/press-release/nyc-mayor-eric-adams-signs-sweet-truth-act. Accessed September 30, 2024.
14. Kaplan S, White JS, Madsen KA, Basu S, Villas-Boas SB, Schillinger D. Evaluation of changes in prices and purchases following implementation of sugar-sweetened beverage taxes across the US. *JAMA Health Forum.* 2024;5(1):e234737. https://doi.org/10.1001/jamahealthforum.2023.4737
15. Young DR, Hedderson MM, Sidell MA, et al. City-level sugar-sweetened beverage taxes and youth body mass index percentile. *JAMA Netw Open.* 2024;7(7):e2424822. https://doi.org/10.1001/jamanetworkopen.2024.24822
16. Kick Big Soda Out of Sport. July 2024. Available at: https://www.kickbigsodaout.org. Accessed September 30, 2024.
17. The Coca-Cola Company. "It's magic when the world comes together": athletes and fans alike embrace global Coca-Cola campaign for Paris 2024 [media release]. July 8, 2024. Available at: https://www.coca-colacompany.com/media-center/its-magic-when-the-world-comes-together-paris2024. Accessed September 30, 2024.

A Treasure Trove Inventory of Sugar-Sweetened Beverage Policies in the United States, 2014–2023

Eric Crosbie, PhD, MA, and Laura Schmidt, PhD, MSW, MPH

ABOUT THE AUTHORS

Eric Crosbie is with the School of Public Health and the Ozmen Institute for Global Studies, University of Nevada, Reno. Laura Schmidt is with the Philip R. Lee Institute for Health Policy Studies, and the Department of Humanities and Social Sciences, University of California, San Francisco.

See also State Laws Targeting Marginalized Groups, pp. 1322–1364.

AJPH December 2024, Vol. 114, No. 12

In this issue of *AJPH*, Davis et al. (p. 1344) map a sustained burst of public health policies regulating sugar-sweetened beverages (SSBs) between 2014 and 2023 that has swept across state, local, and tribal jurisdictions in the United States. This pattern of policy innovation highlights the increased demand for SSB regulations owing to the growing awareness that SSBs are the leading source of dietary added sugars[1] and a steady drumbeat of new publications that call out SSB consumption as a risk factor for cardiometabolic diseases such as type 2 diabetes, dental caries, obesity, and premature mortality.[2] The decade of policy innovation described by Davis et al. kicked off with the first SSB excise taxes ("soda taxes") in Berkeley, California, and the Navajo Nation in 2014—a strategy that now has a robust evidence base showing measurable impacts on SSB sales, childhood obesity, and key disease endpoints, such as gestational diabetes.[3] Proceeds of these soda taxes have been funneled into health and equity programs (e.g., safe drinking water availability, universal prekindergarten), while emboldening further local innovations in healthy retail policies, menu labeling, and growing momentum toward front-of-package nutrition warning labels in the United States.[4]

A key element of the inventory of Davis et al. is its coverage of SSB policies over time, which helps to identify and trace trends and patterns across multiple policy areas and jurisdictions. Examining SSB policies over time reveals how policies with limited evidence of effectiveness (e.g., limited compliance and behavior change with healthy beverage default laws regarding children's meals) prove easier to pass compared with other policies. Although policymakers may earn quick political victories, most local and state policies may not effectively reduce SSB consumption. By contrast, taxation is one of the most effective strategies for reducing SSB consumption, and it is notable that this strategy has been one of the most aggressively fought by the SSB industry—so much so that industry actors have battled to repeal soda taxes even after they have been passed and enacted for years.[5] Researchers and advocates should double down on building the evidence base on the SSB policies that are the most effective and should actively disseminate this knowledge to support the hard work of optimizing policy for true public health impact.

The inventory of Davis et al. also cultivates a better understanding of the overall trajectories of success in policy innovation and where we are in this process for a given type of policy. Consider the case of SSB warning labels, which are particularly effective for mitigating SSB-related harms[6] and currently face an uphill climb toward enactment.[7] The data of Davis et al. suggest that, to become successfully enacted on a widespread basis, warning labels will require multiple running starts, by multiple jurisdictions, before gaining solid traction in the United States. However, the process is clearly under way: the first major SSB warning label policy was passed into law in San Francisco, California, in 2015, alongside a governmental procurement ban on SSBs[8] and a soda tax proposal.

In 2019, *American Beverage Association (ABA) et al. v City & County of San Francisco*, the trade organization representing the SSB industry, successfully blocked the policy because of the size of the required warning and indicated, without ruling definitively, that words such as "type 2" diabetes and "may" could be needed in the text to make it factually accurate.[9] Industry opposes SSB warning labels and aggressively acts to block, weaken, and delay these policies precisely because they are highly effective tools for reducing consumption.[10]

The inventory suggests that it will likely require more valiant efforts such as San Francisco's, even if they fail at enactment, before we can see widespread enactment and diffusion of this evidence-based policy intervention. Part of this approach will be introducing and reintroducing similar and refined policy proposals to force the judicial system to assess the legality of such policies across various jurisdictions. Once legally tested and defended, these rulings could provide important legal support for widespread adoption.

Public health advocates and researchers are often too reactive in responding to threats from powerful health-harming industries, such as the alcohol, tobacco, and food and beverage industries,[11] and the Davis et al. inventory can assist the field to become more proactive by monitoring legislative activity and industry interference. In 2018, the California state legislature was essentially blackmailed by the American Beverage Association in a last-ditch effort to support a state law that preempted any locality in California from enacting SSB taxes through 2030.[5] Similar sneaky and quick state preemptive efforts have succeeded in Arizona, Michigan, and Washington, which have seemed to succeed in preventing the diffusion of these policies throughout the United States.[11] This inventory provides further evidence of this by showing that the speed of new local soda tax laws slowed after 2017, when state preemption efforts picked up speed. Inventories such as this one are essential to preventing preemption and enabling the spread of local SSB taxes. Otherwise, local soda taxes could face the same fate as local smoke-free policies in the United States, where once state preemption was enacted, it took on average 11 years to repeal these policies.[10]

In developing the first comprehensive inventory of nearly 400 SSB policies in the United States, Davis et al. have done a service to the field. The utility of such a comprehensive resource for researchers, policymakers, advocates, public health officials, and community-based organizations will be maximized for population health impact by making it available online and regularly updated. To do so, we should consider modeling this effort on the highly successful Alcohol Policy Information System sponsored by the National Institute on Alcohol Abuse and Alcoholism (https://alcoholpolicy.niaaa.nih.gov), which for decades has provided the alcohol field with a centralized repository of policy information. For researchers, such an online repository would promote important comparative designs such as why some jurisdictions enact taxes and others do not and what the comparative health benefits of local and state policies are. For health advocates, it provides a comprehensive resource of direct Web links to policies and a policy's history assisting with the creation and development of SSB policies. For policymakers, it offers insights into the various facilitators and barriers to policy development and diffusion. AJPH

CORRESPONDENCE

Correspondence should be sent to Eric Crosbie, PhD, Associate Professor, University of Nevada Reno, 1664 Virginia St, Reno, NV 89557 (e-mail: ecrosbie@unr.edu). Reprints can be ordered at https://www.ajph.org by clicking the "Reprints" link.

PUBLICATION INFORMATION

Full Citation: Crosbie E, Schmidt L. A treasure trove inventory of sugar-sweetened beverage policies in the United States, 2014–2023. *Am J Public Health*. 2024;114(12):1326–1327.

Acceptance Date: September 21, 2024.

DOI: https://doi.org/10.2105/AJPH.2024.307881

ORCID iD:

Eric Crosbie https://orcid.org/0000-0002-6219-298X

CONTRIBUTORS

The authors contributed equally to this editorial.

CONFLICTS OF INTEREST

The authors have no conflicts of interest to declare.

REFERENCES

1. Drewnowski A, Rehm CD. Consumption of added sugars among US children and adults by food purchase location and food source. *Am J Clin Nutr*. 2014;100(3):901–907. https://doi.org/10.3945/ajcn.114.089458
2. Malik VS, Hu FB. The role of sugar-sweetened beverages in the global epidemics of obesity and chronic diseases. *Nat Rev Endocrinol*. 2022;18(4):205–218. https://doi.org/10.1038/s41574-021-00627-6
3. Jackson KE, Hamad R, Karasek D, White JS. Sugar-sweetened beverage taxes and perinatal health: a quasi-experimental study. *Am J Prev Med*. 2023;65(3):366–376. [Corrigendum in: *Am J Prev Med*. 2024;67(1):167–174. https://doi.org/10.1016/j.amepre.2024.02.008]. https://doi.org/10.1016/j.amepre.2023.03.016
4. Krieger J, Magee K, Hennings T, Schoof J, Madsen KA. How sugar-sweetened beverage tax revenues are being used in the United States. *Prev Med Rep*. 2021;23:101388. https://doi.org/10.1016/j.pmedr.2021.101388
5. Crosbie E, Pomeranz JL, Wright KE, Hoeper S, Schmidt L. State preemption: an emerging threat to local sugar-sweetened beverage taxation. *Am J Public Health*. 2021;111(4):677–686. https://doi.org/10.2105/AJPH.2020.306062
6. An R, Liu J, Liu R, Barker AR, Figueroa RB, McBride TD. Impact of sugar-sweetened beverage warning labels on consumer behaviors: a systematic review and meta-analysis. *Am J Prev Med*. 2021;60(1):115–126. https://doi.org/10.1016/j.amepre.2020.07.003
7. Schillinger D, Jacobson MF. Science and public health on trial: warning notices on advertisements for sugary drinks. *JAMA*. 2016;316(15):1545–1546. https://doi.org/10.1001/jama.2016.10516
8. Pomeranz JL, Mozaffarian D, Micha R. Sugar-sweetened beverage warning policies in the broader legal context: health and safety warning laws and the First Amendment. *Am J Prev Med*. 2020;58(6):783–788. https://doi.org/10.1016/j.amepre.2020.01.006
9. Popova L, Nonnemaker J, Taylor N, Bradfield B, Kim A. Warning labels on sugar-sweetened beverages: an eye tracking approach. *Am J Health Behav*. 2019;43(2):406–419. https://doi.org/10.5993/AJHB.43.2.16
10. Crosbie E, Schmidt LA. Preemption in tobacco control: a framework for other areas of public health. *Am J Public Health*. 2020;110(3):345–350. https://doi.org/10.2105/AJPH.2019.305473
11. Crosbie E, Schillinger D, Schmidt LA. State preemption to prevent local taxation of sugar-sweetened beverages. *JAMA Intern Med*. 2019;179(3):291–292. https://doi.org/10.1001/jamainternmed.2018.7770

All Hands on Deck: Addressing Obstacles to Applying an Intersectionality Framework in Health Research

Danielle M. Crookes, DrPH

ABOUT THE AUTHOR

Danielle M. Crookes is with the Department of Public Health and Health Sciences, Bouvé College of Health Sciences, and the Department of Sociology and Anthropology, College of Social Sciences and Humanities, Northeastern University, Boston, MA.

See also State Laws Targeting Marginalized Groups, pp. 1322–1364.

AJPH December 2024, Vol. 114, No. 12

In "The Synergistic Health Threats of State Laws Targeting Marginalized Groups in the United States," Underhill et al. (p. 1335) issue a call based on the intersectionality framework to scholars to examine the effects of laws in multiple domains on the health of people belonging to multiple marginalized groups. Here, I amplify that call by focusing on two areas where epidemiologists and other quantitative health scholars can also advance the application of intersectionality theory in health research.

Intersectionality traces back to Black feminist scholarship of the 1970s through the 1990s, but it was not rapidly adopted and adapted by social science and public health disciplines until the mid-2000s.[1] Despite the wide embrace of intersectionality, scholars across disciplines, including mine (i.e., epidemiology), either continue to approach health in a compartmentalized way (as Underhill et al. highlight in their study) or grapple with how to appropriately implement and apply the intersectionality framework in health research.[2] I suggest that emphasis on precision in causal inference and the relative infancy of measuring systems of oppression (e.g., sexism, racism, ableism) within domains contribute to slower advances in the application of intersectionality in health research and that opportunities exist to make further strides.

PRECISION IN CAUSAL INFERENCE

Epidemiologists and other quantitative health researchers are trained in causal methods to identify causes of disease and to estimate causal effects of different exposures on outcomes (e.g., in epidemiology, methods are centered on the sufficient component cause model and the potential outcomes model[3]). Epidemiologists are trained to first envision well-defined interventions and identify specific combinations of exposures (i.e., component causes) and then address confounding, measurement bias, and selection bias in our studies to yield unbiased estimates of causal effects. In this process, we attempt to strip away all other possible explanations that could muddy the exposure–outcome effect estimates.

This approach benefits both causal inference and the identification of specific actionable interventions, such as policies, but is also limited in its ability to address the complexity of the policy environment. As Underhill et al. highlight, others have documented that discriminatory laws cooccur and often do so in geographic and temporal patterns, making it more challenging to identify the health effects of single policies. The recent increase in studies on policies' impacts on health prompted Matthay et al. to examine social policy cooccurrence and to identify potential threats to causal inference.[4] They demonstrated that social policies within domains (e.g., firearms, cannabis, social welfare) rarely occur in isolation and that considerable challenges exist in estimating their individual effects with precision, let alone in combination with policies across domains. This desire to improve causal inference about a single policy or specific policy clusters holds value both for causal inference and for policymaking, but it also reinforces compartmentalization. The predominant use of methods to isolate policy effects (e.g., adjusting for cooccurring policies in models, selecting less correlated policy exposure measures[5]) thwarts examination of systems of oppression across domains and ignores the experiences of people affected by multiple policies across systems.

Epidemiologic methods are currently limited in their ability to examine the complexity of interacting systems of oppression, but the field of systems science was founded to understand the interaction between multiple variables and changes in systems over time. Opportunities exist to bridge the gaps between systems science and epidemiology and to incorporate perspectives from each field into the study of health.[6] Those interested in applying the intersectionality framework to health equity can benefit from training in both traditional causal inference methods and systems science methods or from collaborations with scholars in both fields to develop novel, stronger analytic approaches for understanding the health effects of these interacting systems of oppression.

MEASURING SYSTEMS OF OPPRESSION

Even though the intersectionality framework has existed for some time, putting this framework into practice and measuring the systems and institutions that drive health inequities is still relatively new. Domain-specific advancement in measurement of these systems may be necessary before analyses across domains can be successfully conducted. For example, the study of racism has grown over time, beginning with studies of interpersonal and internalized racism and expanding to studies of structural racism. Over time, the definition of structural racism has also evolved and so have the measures that scholars have used to apply it in their research.[7]

For example, as the definition of structural racism has evolved (e.g., recently defined as the "totality of ways in which societies foster racial discrimination through mutually reinforcing systems of housing, education, employment, earnings, benefits, credit, media, health care, and criminal justice"[8(p1453)]), more complex measures, such as indexes of structural racism indicators (e.g., Black–White inequalities in homeownership or college education, laws that disadvantage people of color), have been developed.[7] These indexes capture the complexity of structural racism better than unidimensional measures such as residential segregation.

Similar growth has occurred in the study of immigrant health. Over the past few decades, there has been increased examination of the health effects of immigration policies at federal, state, and local levels. Although several studies in this area have focused on single policies (e.g., Deferred Action for Childhood Arrivals, 287(g) agreements), a few studies have begun to use indexes of policies across health care, mobility, and language access for capturing the multiple ways newly arrived and undocumented immigrants' rights, protections, and lives are governed.[9] The ongoing growth in the measurement of racism and xenophobia has advanced research focused on the health effects of multiple, interacting forces within these specific systems of oppression. Still, the conceptualization of these systems of oppression continues to be siloed[10] and thus does not address the interaction between these systems of oppression that is required under the intersectionality framework.

As advancement in the measurement of specific systems of oppression continues, it will be necessary to go beyond acknowledging that other systems of oppression exist and begin to examine how they interact to address the health of people holding multiple marginalized identities. Recently, Homan et al. proposed a structural intersectionality approach to better conceptualize and measure joint effects of multiple systems of oppression on health.[11] This proposed approach explicitly brings intersectionality back to the front and center and, coupled with the advancements in measurement of domain-specific systems of oppression, holds promise for encouraging collaborative work to advance the application of the intersectionality framework in health research.

As Underhill et al. suggest, a multilateral effort is required to address the effects of intersecting systems of oppression that threaten the health of multiply marginalized groups. They demonstrate how public health law scholars can better incorporate the intersectionality framework in their identification and analysis of laws. I similarly implore epidemiologists and others involved in quantitative health research to reexamine the limitations of our current approaches and focus on ways that we can contribute to advancing the application of intersectionality in health research. AJPH

CORRESPONDENCE

Correspondence should be sent to Danielle M. Crookes, Assistant Professor, Northeastern University, 360 Huntington Ave, Boston, MA 02115 (e-mail: d.crookes@northeastern.edu). Reprints can be ordered at https://www.ajph.org by clicking the "Reprints" link.

PUBLICATION INFORMATION

Full Citation: Crookes DM. All hands on deck: addressing obstacles to applying an intersectionality framework in health research. *Am J Public Health*. 2024;114(12):1328–1330.

Acceptance Date: September 21, 2024.

DOI: https://doi.org/10.2105/AJPH.2024.307882

ORCID iD:

Danielle M. Crookes https://orcid.org/0000-0002-6834-1835

ACKNOWLEDGMENTS

I thank the historical and current scholars of intersectionality, structural racism, and immigrant health for their personal and professional labor in conducting the research on which these comments are based.

CONFLICTS OF INTEREST

The author has no conflicts of interest to declare.

REFERENCES

1. Collins PH. Intersectionality's definitional dilemmas. *Annu Rev Sociol.* 2015;41:1–20. https://doi.org/10.1146/annurev-soc-073014-112142
2. Guan A, Thomas M, Vittinghoff E, Bowleg L, Mangurian C, Wesson P. An investigation of quantitative methods for assessing intersectionality in health research: a systematic review. *SSM Popul Health.* 2021;16:100977. https://doi.org/10.1016/j.ssmph.2021.100977
3. Flanders WD. On the relationship of sufficient component cause models with potential outcome (counterfactual) models. *Eur J Epidemiol.* 2006;21(12):847–853. https://doi.org/10.1007/s10654-006-9048-3
4. Matthay EC, Hagan E, Joshi S, et al. The revolution will be hard to evaluate: how co-occurring policy changes affect research on the health effects of social policies. *Epidemiol Rev.* 2021;43(1):19–32. https://doi.org/10.1093/epirev/mxab009
5. Matthay EC, Gottlieb LM, Rehkopf D, Tan ML, Vlahov D, Glymour MM. What to do when everything happens at once: analytic approaches to estimate the health effects of co-occurring social policies. *Epidemiol Rev.* 2021;43(1):33–47. https://doi.org/10.1093/epirev/mxab005
6. Cerdá M, Keyes KM. Systems modeling to advance the promise of data science in epidemiology. *Am J Epidemiol.* 2019;188(5):862–865. https://doi.org/10.1093/aje/kwy262
7. Dean LT, Thorpe RJ Jr. What structural racism is (or is not) and how to measure it: clarity for public health and medical researchers. *Am J Epidemiol.* 2022;191(9):1521–1526. https://doi.org/10.1093/aje/kwac112
8. Bailey ZD, Krieger N, Agénor M, Graves J, Linos N, Bassett MT. Structural racism and health inequities in the USA: evidence and interventions. *Lancet.* 2017;389(10077):1453–1463. https://doi.org/10.1016/S0140-6736(17)30569-X
9. Crookes DM, Stanhope KK, Suglia SF. Immigrant-related policies and the health outcomes of Latinx adults in the United States: a systematic review. *Epidemiology.* 2022;33(4):593–605. https://doi.org/10.1097/EDE.0000000000001480
10. Joseph T, Golash-Boza T. Double consciousness in the 21st century: Du Boisian theory and the problem of racialized legal status. *Soc Sci.* 2021;10(9):345. https://doi.org/10.3390/socsci10090345
11. Homan P, Brown TH, King B. Structural intersectionality as a new direction for health disparities research. *J Health Soc Behav.* 2021;62(3):350–370. https://doi.org/10.1177/00221465211032947

The Return of Jim Crow: Government Discrimination Against Women, LGBTQIA+ Individuals, and Racial/Ethnic Minority Individuals

Ruqaiijah Yearby, JD, MPH

ABOUT THE AUTHOR

Ruqaiijah Yearby is with the Moritz College of Law and the Department of Health Services Management and Policy, College of Public Health, The Ohio State University, Columbus.

See also State Laws Targeting Marginalized Groups, pp. 1322–1364.

Within the past 14 years, Congress has enacted prohibitions against sex discrimination in health care, the Supreme Court has granted employment protections to lesbian, gay, bisexual, transgender, queer or questioning, intersex, asexual or ally, and other (LGBTQIA+) individuals, and more than 300 US localities have declared racism a public health crisis. These governmental actions sought to make the promise of equality found in the 14th Amendment of the US Constitution a reality for women as well as LGBTQIA+ and racial/ethnic minority individuals.

However, since 2022, some states not only have begun to enact laws targeting these groups, as discussed in this issue of *AJPH* by Underhill et al. (p. 1335), but have also sought to eliminate civil rights protections for women and LGBTQIA+ and racial/ethnic minority individuals.[1] Both actions evidence a return to the discrimination of the Jim Crow era, when the government mandated and financially supported the unequal treatment of racial/ethnic minority individuals, women, and LGBTQIA+ individuals. This will harm individuals of all gender identities, sexual orientations, races, and ethnicities.[2–4]

THE PROMISE OF EQUALITY

The Patient Protection and Affordable Care Act of 2010 (ACA) increased access to health insurance for all individuals.[5] Section 1557 of the ACA expanded protections against racial discrimination and prohibited sex discrimination by those receiving federal financial assistance, which includes health care institutions, providers, and insurance companies. Moreover, the ACA barred nongroup and individually purchased insurance plans from "charging women higher premiums than men for the same level of coverage (gender rating) or from disqualifying women from coverage because they had certain preexisting medical conditions, including pregnancy."[6] The regulations enforcing Section 1557 of the ACA included LGBTQIA+ individuals under these sex nondiscrimination protections.[7] As a result of the ACA, racial/ethnic inequities in insurance coverage decreased, and just as progress stalled many localities began to declare racism as a public health crisis (RPHC).[2,8]

Between 2014 and 2021, 313 localities declared RPHC to decrease racial inequities and increase equity by addressing past and modern-day instances of racial discrimination. For example, Amherst, Massachusetts, declared RPHC and enacted a reparations fund, whereas the RPHC declarations by Lansing, Michigan, Austin, Texas, and Louisville, Kentucky, acknowledged the government's role in supporting racially segregated housing.[8] Many of these declarations noted that racial discrimination continued to limit racial/ethnic minority individuals' equality and were accompanied by plans to address this inequality. However, the protections and benefits of the ACA and RPHC declarations are being eroded by states that are targeting women, LGBTQIA+ individuals, and racial/ethnic minority individuals, which is reminiscent of the Jim Crow era. Table 1 shows the current and Jim Crow era discriminatory policies and actions adopted by states.

THE JIM CROW ERA

During the Jim Crow era (1877–1968), also known as the Jane Crow era, the government mandated and financially supported the unequal treatment of women as well as LGBTQIA+ and racial/ethnic minority individuals. They also supported neutral laws and policies, which had a disproportionately

TABLE 1— Current and Jim Crow Era Discriminatory Policies and Actions: United States, 1877–2024

	Current (2022–Present)			Jim Crow Era (1877–1968)		
States	Abortion (25 States)	Anti-LGBTQIA+ (17 States)	Petition Against Title VI Disparate Impact (23 States)	Abortion (50 States)	Sodomy Laws Targeting LGBTQIA+ Individuals (21 States)	Hill-Burton Unequal Health Care Facilities (14 States)
Alabama	X	X	X	X	X	X
Arkansas	X	X	X	X	X	
Florida	X	X	X	X	X	X
Georgia	X	X	X	X	X	X
Idaho	X		X	X		
Indiana	X	X	X	X		
Iowa	X	X	X	X		
Kansas			X	X	X	
Kentucky	X	X	X	X	X	X
Louisiana	X	X		X		X
Maryland				X	X	X
Mississippi	X	X	X	X	X	X
Missouri	X		X	X	X	X
Montana		X	X	X	X	
Nebraska	X	X	X	X		
Nevada				X	X	
North Carolina	X	X		X	X	X
North Dakota	X	X	X	X	X	
Oklahoma	X	X	X	X	X	X
Pennsylvania	X			X	X	
South Carolina	X		X	X		X
South Dakota	X		X	X	X	
Tennessee	X		X	X	X	X
Texas	X	X	X	X	X	
Utah	X	X	X	X	X	
Virginia			X	X	X	X
Washington				X	X	
West Virginia	X		X	X		X
Wyoming	X		X	X		

Note. LGBTQIA+ = lesbian, gay, bisexual, transgender, queer or questioning, intersex, asexual or ally, and others.
Source. Data for the Jim Crow era were compiled from Planned Parenthood Action Fund,[9] American Civil Liberties Union,[10] and Yearby.[11] Table compiled from the Center for Reproductive Rights,[12] Underhill et al. (p. 1335), and the State of Florida Attorney General.[1]

harmful effect on these groups. For instance, by 1910, every state had outlawed abortions, with some exceptions for saving the pregnant person's life. The decision to grant these exceptions was left to physicians, who at that time were predominantly (95%) male.[9] These abortion bans were supported by White male legislators "as a way to get upper-class White women to have more children"[9] in response to an increase in immigration.[10] In 1930 almost one in five maternal deaths was connected to illegal abortion.[9]

In the late 1960s, some state legislatures began to rewrite sodomy laws to apply to only gay people, and some state agencies and courts began to apply sodomy laws to only gay people.[10] These laws were used to deny gay parents' custody of their children and prevent LGBTQIA+ individuals from obtaining jobs.[10] The government also adopted laws and policies that mandated and supported racial/ethnic minority individuals' unequal access to health care.

In 1935, Congress enacted the Social Security Act, which provided federal funding to private institutions for the care of the elderly. At that time a majority of elderly racial/ethnic minority individuals received their care in public institutions, which were prohibited from receiving this funding.[11] The Hill–Burton Act (i.e., the 1946 Hospital Survey and Construction Act) provided federal funding for the construction of public hospitals, creating our current hospital system, but Section 622(f) of the act explicitly allowed states to racially segregate hospitals. As a result, 14 states constructed separate and unequal health care facilities for Black patients.[11]

States also allowed White-only hospitals to limit medical staff privileges to those who were board certified and members of a medical society. Because most racial/ethnic minority physicians were denied access to specialty training in hospitals and membership in medical societies, this race-neutral policy prevented racial/ethnic minority physicians from obtaining staff privileges at White-only hospitals, which also meant their patients were banned from these hospitals.[11] Research shows that Black infant deaths were higher in states with Jim Crow policies and that this disparity shrank with the enactment of civil rights laws.[13] Several civil rights laws were enacted in the 1960s; however, currently some states are targeting and seeking to eliminate these civil rights protections for women as well as LGBTQIA+ and racial/ethnic minority individuals.

THE RETURN TO JIM CROW SINCE 2022

Since the Supreme Court overturned *Roe v Wade* in 2022, 25 states have enacted laws that significantly impair or totally ban access to abortions.[12] Similar to the abortion bans during the Jim Crow era, many of these recent bans have been enacted by legislatures that are mostly male, and some of these legislatures have called the bans a "victory for White life" in response to increased immigration.[14] Research has shown that there are higher death rates among all women of reproductive age as well as higher rates of maternal and infant mortality among all racial groups in states that have total bans or restrictions on abortions.[4] These states also have greater racial/ethnic inequities in their health care systems, including inequities in maternal and infant mortality rates.[4]

During the same time, some states also began enacting laws targeting LGBTQIA+ individuals, including limiting access to gender-affirming care for transgender youths. Many of these same states changed sodomy laws in the 1960s to apply to only LGBTQIA+ individuals. Survey data have shown an association between these laws targeting LGBTQIA+ youths and an increase in LGBTQIA+ youths considering committing suicide.[3] In fact, almost one in three LGBTQIA+ youths have said their mental health was worse because of anti-LGBTQIA+ laws and policies.[9]

Additionally, 23 attorneys general have filed a petition for rule making with the Environmental Protection Agency to eliminate regulations prohibiting disparate impact discrimination.[1] Notably, 11 of the 23 states challenging these civil rights protections were the same states that constructed racially separate and unequal health care facilities during Jim Crow. The language of Title VI of the Civil Rights Act of 1964 is based, in large part, on a successful case that challenged disparate treatment and disparate impact discrimination in health care.[11] Moreover, since 1966, when the Title VI regulations were finalized, the federal government has used the regulations to address disparate impact discrimination.

For example, in the 1970s, the US Department of Health and Human Services used the regulations to stop Barnes Hospital (St. Louis, MO) from racially segregating obstetrics–gynecology patients. Specifically, Black and White obstetrics–gynecology patients at Barnes Hospital were racially segregated using a race-neutral policy.[15] A civil rights complaint was filed with the Department of Health and Human Services, who ruled against Barnes Hospital and put an end to racial segregation in obstetrics–gynecology services at Barnes Hospital. This ruling and racial integration would not have been possible if the government had not been able to address disparate impact discrimination. Yet, in their 2024 petition, the attorneys general argue that enforcing the regulations require government officials to adopt racial quotas, which harm White individuals. Contrary to these unsupported claims, the enforcement of disparate impact regulations do not result in racial quotas; instead, they allow the government to stop government-sponsored racially segregated health care.

CONCLUSIONS

Some of the same states that were ardent supporters of Jim Crow discrimination are not only enacting laws that target women, LGBTQIA+ individuals, and racial/ethnic minority individuals but also actively trying to eliminate civil rights protections for these groups. These actions are often supported by the same discriminatory rhetoric used during the Jim Crow era. Research has already begun to show that these actions harm women, LGBTQIA+ individuals, and racial/ethnic minority individuals, as well as individuals of all races, ethnicities, gender identities, and sexual orientations.[2–4] Thus, the time has come to counter these state actions by working to make the promise of equality found in the 14th Amendment of the US Constitution a reality for everyone.

AJPH

CORRESPONDENCE

Correspondence should be sent to Ruqaiijah Yearby, JD, MPH, The Ohio State University, Moritz College of Law, 55 W. 12th Ave, Columbus, OH 43210 (e-mail: yearby.1@osu.edu). Reprints can be ordered at https://www.ajph.org by clicking the "Reprints" link.

PUBLICATION INFORMATION

Full Citation: Yearby R. The return of Jim Crow: government discrimination against women, LGBTQIA+ individuals, and racial/ethnic minority individuals. *Am J Public Health*. 2024;114(12): 1331–1334.

Acceptance Date: September 26, 2024.

DOI: https://doi.org/10.2105/AJPH.2024.307884

ORCID iD:

Ruqaiijah Yearby https://orcid.org/0000-0002-2381-9401

CONFLICTS OF INTEREST

The author has no conflicts of interest to disclose.

REFERENCES

1. State of Florida Attorney General. Petition for rulemaking. April 16, 2024. Available at: https://www.myfloridalegal.com/site.s/default/files/2024-04/epa-title-vi-comment-final.pdf. Accessed September 15, 2024.
2. Baumgartner JC, Collins SR, Radley DC, Hayes SL. How the Affordable Care Act has narrowed racial and ethnic disparities in access to health care. January 16, 2020. Available at: https://www.commonwealthfund.org/publications/2020/jan/how-ACA-narrowed-racial-ethnic-disparities-access. Accessed September 15, 2024.
3. Trevor Project. 2023 US National Survey on the Mental Health of LGBTQ Young People. 2023. Available at: https://www.thetrevorproject.org/survey-2023. Accessed September 15, 2024.
4. Declercq E, Barnard-Mayers R, Zephyrin LC, Johnson K. The US maternal health divide: the limited maternal health services and worse outcomes of states proposing new abortion restrictions. December 14, 2022. Available at: https://www.commonwealthfund.org/publications/issue-briefs/2022/dec/us-maternal-health-divide-limited-services-worse-outcomes. Accessed September 15, 2024.
5. Office of the Legislative Counsel. Compilation of Patient Protection and Affordable Care Act. As amended through May 1, 2010. June 10, 2010. Available at: https://housedocs.house.gov/energycommerce/ppacacon.pdf. Accessed September 15, 2024.
6. Kaiser Family Foundation. Women's health insurance coverage. December 13, 2023. Available at: https://www.kff.org/womens-health-policy/fact-sheet/womens-health-insurance-coverage. Accessed September 15, 2024.
7. Baker K. LGBTQ protections in Affordable Care Act Section 1557. *Health Affairs Forefront*. June 6, 2016. Available at: https://doi.org/10.1377/forefront.20160606.055155. Accessed October 3, 2024.
8. Lewis CN, Yearby R, Gibson C, Jaeger AR, Lawson MT. Racism is a public health crisis: how local governments are responding. August 22, 2022. Available at: https://ihje.org/our-work/reports/racism-is-a-public-health-crisis-report-2. Accessed September 15, 2024.
9. Planned Parenthood Action Fund. Historical abortion law timeline: 1850 to today. Available at: https://www.plannedparenthoodaction.org/issues/abortion/abortion-central-history-reproductive-health-care-america/historical-abortion-law-timeline-1850-today. Accessed September 15, 2024.
10. American Civil Liberties Union. Why sodomy laws matter. June 26, 2023. Available at: https://www.aclu.org/documents/why-sodomy-laws-matter. Accessed September 15, 2024.
11. Yearby R. When is a change going to come: separate and unequal treatment in health care fifty years after the Title VI of the Civil Rights Act of 1964. *SMU Law Rev*. 2014;67(2):287–337.
12. Center for Reproductive Rights. After Roe fell: abortion laws by state. Available at: https://reproductiverights.org/maps/abortion-laws-by-state. Accessed September 15, 2024.
13. Krieger N, Chen JT, Coull B, Waterman PD, Beckfield J. The unique impact of abolition of Jim Crow laws on reducing inequities in infant death rates and implications for choice of comparison groups in analyzing societal determinants of health. *Am J Public Health*. 2013;103(12):2234–2244. https://doi.org/10.2105/AJPH.2013.301350
14. Churchwell S. Body politics: the secret history of the US anti-abortion movement. *The Guardian*. July 23, 2022. Available at: https://www.theguardian.com/books/2022/jul/23/body-politics. Accessed September 15, 2024.
15. Saunders PN. Oral history. July 6, 1990. Available at: https://becker.wustl.edu/static-files/arb/016-PC054-WUMCDesegregationHistoryProject/PC054-S12-B01-F27-i01_Paul_N_Saunders_oral_history_transcript.pdf. Accessed September 15, 2024.

The Synergistic Health Threats of State Laws Targeting Marginalized Groups in the United States

Kristen Underhill, DPhil, JD, Valerie A. Earnshaw, PhD, and Kimberly M. Nelson, PhD, MPH

See also State Laws Targeting Marginalized Groups, pp. 1322–1364.

Discriminatory state laws have deleterious effects on the health of socially marginalized groups. Health care clinicians, institutions, researchers, and research funders have tended to view different discriminatory laws in isolation, focusing on particular issues or groups. In contrast, intersectionality calls attention to the overlapping and synergistic systems of oppression that discriminatory legislation promotes or upholds, warranting an integrated analysis of these laws.

In this analytic essay, we assess discriminatory state laws simultaneously and discuss their implications for health care clinicians, institutions, and researchers. We present a multifunctional model of law and population health that describes how discriminatory law affects health outcomes among marginalized groups. We then draw on publicly available legislation trackers to identify 30 states that have enacted legislation since 2020 that targets Black people and other people of color; lesbian, gay, bisexual, and queer people; transgender and nonbinary people; and women and other birthing people.

Finally, we call for a coordinated, multilateral, and forceful effort by health care professionals, institutions, researchers, and research funders to counter these laws and address their predictable health consequences.
(*Am J Public Health*. 2024;114(12):1335–1343. https://doi.org/10.2105/AJPH.2024.307830)

AJPH December 2024, Vol. 114, No. 12

State law in the United States has long played an active part—sometimes a starring role—in maintaining power imbalances by race, ethnicity, sexual orientation, gender identity, and sex. A new surge of discriminatory state legislation in the United States has diminished protections for marginalized social groups, including Black people and other people of color; lesbian, gay, bisexual, and queer (LGBQ) people; transgender people; and women and other people capable of pregnancy. Public health law theory posits that laws have direct and indirect consequences for population health,[1] including the health of marginalized populations.[2] A growing body of research has documented associations between laws that adversely target marginalized populations (i.e., discriminatory laws) and poorer health among members of those groups.[3–5] Building on the legacies of early thinkers in intersectionality, such as bell hooks, Kimberlé Crenshaw, Pauli Murray, W.E.B. Du Bois, James McCune Smith, and members of the Black feminist Combahee River Collective, health inequities research recognizes linkages between discriminatory policies and health of multiply marginalized groups. An intersectionality framework suggests that these laws stem from, and contribute to, overlapping and synergistic systems of marginalization, including but not limited to racism, sexism, heterosexism, and cisgenderism.[6] As these systems interact, discriminatory laws may target more than 1 group at a time or impact people at the intersections of multiple forms of oppression.[6]

These dynamics bolster a theory-driven prediction: when legislation adversely targets a marginalized group, we should anticipate health consequences for that group, for other marginalized groups, and for subgroups that experience multiple forms of structural disadvantage. This analysis considers recent laws targeting Black people and other people of color, LGBQ people, transgender people, and women and other people capable of pregnancy, as illustrative but not exhaustive examples of discriminatory legislation. Given that more than half of US people experience 1 or more of these forms of marginalization, recent discriminatory legislation demands a forceful response not only by policymakers and advocates but also by health care professionals, institutions, researchers, and research funders.

FROM DISCRIMINATORY LAWS TO HEALTH OUTCOMES

Legal epidemiologists have identified multiple pathways connecting law to health.[1,7] Statutes, regulations, and judicial decisions result from complex social and political forces, which exert their own impacts on health and make it difficult to disaggregate the effects of law itself. Some studies therefore use law as an indicator of environment (e.g., a recent review identified 58 studies that use laws to indicate the presence or magnitude of structural stigma targeting LGBQ and transgender people[8]). Other studies focus on the direct and indirect health impacts of laws, which is our focus here. The health impacts of laws might be intended (e.g., laws restricting vaccine exemptions can reduce infectious disease outbreaks[9]) or unintended (e.g., COVID-19 lockdowns were associated with increased drug overdose deaths[10]).

The most prominent framework in public health law research proposes that law simultaneously exerts direct effects on behavior, direct effects on the social and built environment, and indirect effects on behavior via the environment, all of which cumulatively impact population health.[1] This model also recognizes that law can shape social attitudes, including (de)stigmatizing social statuses,[11] and these social attitudes have both direct and indirect impacts on population health.

Stigma—a social process emerging at the co-occurrence of labeling, stereotyping, separation, and discriminatory treatment within a power context—is a "fundamental cause" of health inequities affecting marginalized populations.[12,13] We suggest that discriminatory laws are structural-level manifestations of stigma that are likely to impact public health through multiple pathways. Specifically, we illustrate 2 mutually reinforcing functions of law in Figure 1: compliance and expressive functions. In its compliance function, law requires, subsidizes, licenses, burdens, or prohibits behaviors (e.g., a "bathroom bill" prohibits transgender people from using gender-congruent public bathrooms). In its expressive function, law codifies values regarding what,

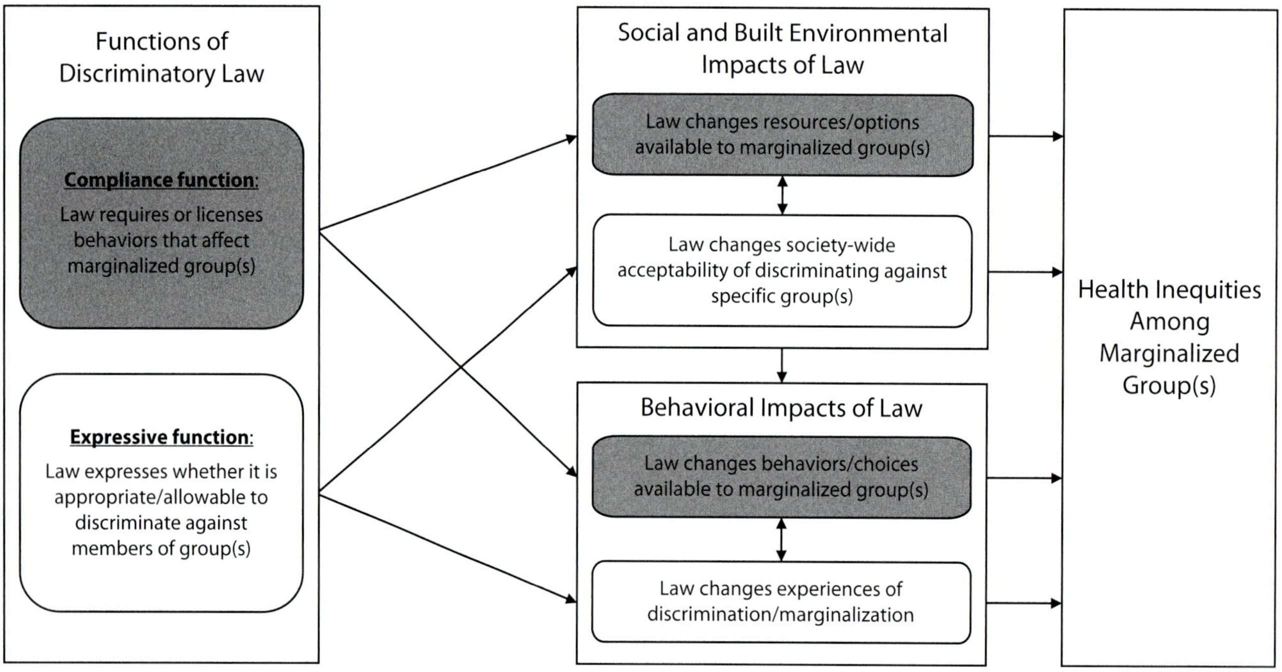

FIGURE 1— A Multifunctional Model of Discriminatory Law and Population Health

Note. This figure develops a logic model for public health law research to demonstrate 2 separate but linked functions of law. In its compliance function, law sets forth prohibitions, mandates, costs, and incentives for behavior. In its expressive function, law encodes messages about social values, which change or reinforce social norms. Laws work through both of these pathways to shape resources, social and built environments, behavioral options, and experiences for members of marginalized groups.

and who, deserves attention, dignity, respect, autonomy, protection, and care. Furthermore, through its expressive function, law takes a position on whether it is appropriate and allowable to treat a specific social group differently—for instance, a bathroom bill expresses that it is appropriate to deny transgender people something that cisgender people have (i.e., access to public restrooms that accord with their gender identity).

Both the compliance and expressive functions of law can lead to environmental and behavioral impacts, and these pathways are mutually reinforcing. We trace the compliance function first. Through the compliance function, discriminatory laws affect the environment by changing the options or resources available to a marginalized group (e.g., bathroom bills decrease the availability of gender-congruent public facilities for transgender individuals). The compliance function also affects behavior as people adjust to the legal change. Law can drive behavior among members of the marginalized population (e.g., bathroom bills require transgender people to avoid bathrooms or to use facilities where they may experience harassment, abuse, and unwanted disclosure). Law can also influence behavior by other actors (e.g., in states with bathroom bills, public facilities or bystanders enforce the exclusion of transgender people from gender-congruent facilities). Where laws operate to reduce access to resources, such as access to health care or economic opportunity, these mechanisms can inflict material deprivation and consequent harms experienced by the target population.

The expressive function of law also has environmental and behavioral impacts. Discriminatory laws affect social norms, which are part of the social environment. Because discriminatory laws license or require adverse treatment of a marginalized group, they express and elevate the social norm that it is appropriate to disadvantage group members (e.g., bathroom bills express support for treating transgender people with less dignity and regard than cisgender people). The expressive functions of discriminatory laws can also affect behaviors and experiences among the marginalized group and others. For people who are aware of the law (e.g., transgender people who learn that the legislature has barred them from gender-congruent public bathrooms), the enactment of a discriminatory statute is inherently stigmatizing, with corollary consequences for health, even if the law is not enforced. As the law is implemented, the expressive function also facilitates or provides for individual behaviors that label, separate, and discriminate against the targeted group (e.g., bathroom bills empower people to question or challenge bathroom users whose gender presentation does not match sex stereotypes). This, in turn, leads people in the targeted group to experience more discrimination, stress, and resource scarcity.

Because powerful social institutions and actors take direction from law, the expressive impacts of discriminatory laws can also spread throughout the social environment, "spilling over" beyond the specific prohibitions or requirements of the law. In this way, the expressive impacts of a discriminatory law can be even more powerful than the law's compliance impacts. A bathroom bill in public facilities, for example, can encourage private facilities to enact or maintain similar policies (spilling over to a different setting), or it can support discrimination against cisgender people who do not conform to expected gender appearances (spilling over to a different group).[14,15] It may be enforced more frequently against transgender individuals with additional marginalized identities, like transgender women or transgender people of color (intersectional harms against multiply marginalized groups). Because bathroom bills allow differential treatment of transgender individuals, they can be cited to support practices that exclude transgender people—or cisgender people who do not conform to gender stereotypes—in nonbathroom settings (spilling over to a different group and a different setting). A bill in one state can reduce political or popular support for gender-inclusive practices in neighboring towns across the state line (spilling over to a different jurisdiction). Bathroom bills also strengthen ideas of gender essentialism and "benevolent" sexism that are already linked to harmful outcomes for transgender people and cisgender women and girls.[16]

In these ways, the effects of a discriminatory law can reach beyond its intended population and jurisdiction, escalating the society-wide processes of labeling, stereotyping, separation, material deprivation, and discrimination that harm the health of devalued groups.[13] And although laws are themselves the product of many different forces (e.g., politics, resources, procedural options, interest group pressures), increased stigma can foster a supportive public environment for future discriminatory legislation. Importantly, this multifunctional model of the health impacts of discriminatory law can apply to any nation, state, or municipality with laws that marginalize (or allow marginalization of) a social group.

DISCRIMINATORY LAWS AND INTERSECTIONALITY

Laws burdening different marginalized groups occur in every state, and they tend to cluster within states,[17] in part because many jurisdictions maintain a fairly continuous orientation toward policy over time.[18] Intersectionality—a framework rooted in Black feminist theory[19,20]—emphasizes that systems of oppression, including stigma, are interlocking and synergistic.[6] Indeed, while methods for intersectionality health research are developing rapidly, systematic reviews now identify hundreds of studies documenting differential health burdens (e.g., chronic conditions, hypertension, sexually transmitted infections, suicidal ideation, substance use) among people who hold multiple socially marginalized identities.[21,22] Applied to discriminatory law, intersectionality suggests that co-occurring discriminatory laws are likely to have differential and possibly compounding effects specifically on the health of multiply marginalized people. In any jurisdiction where laws burden multiple marginalized populations simultaneously, these policies can work in concert to harm the health of individuals and groups. For individuals who experience multiple forms of discrimination (e.g., Black cisgender women, Latine transgender men, sexual minoritized women) adverse state laws can interact to produce synergistic harms.[23]

Consider, for example, a North Dakota high-school student who identifies as a Black transgender girl. Since 2020, the state legislature has passed anti–critical race theory and antitransgender laws, each targeting a different aspect of her social identity. She will experience direct consequences of each law—schools where educators cannot provide "instruction relating to critical race theory" (HB 1508 [2021]), health systems in which she cannot access gender-affirming care (HB 1254 [2023]), and an extracurricular environment where she cannot participate in student athletics (HB 1249 [2023]). These barriers can increase experiences of exclusion and isolation, while the laws convey a cumulative message that she is less valued. The laws also express and sanction the general principles that it is acceptable to withhold medical care from transgender people, limit social participation by transgender people, or forbid classroom instruction that recognizes structural racism or includes central intellectual contributions by Black people and other people of color. All of these dynamics can amplify stigma and discrimination as part of the general social environment.

There are at least 3 implications of applying an intersectionality framework to understanding how discriminatory laws impact health outcomes. First, as mentioned previously, individuals belonging to multiple marginalized groups may be targeted by multiple discriminatory laws. Second, discriminatory laws may target more than 1 marginalized group, shifting power and opportunities away from multiple groups simultaneously. For example, Legislative Bill 574 in Nebraska (2023) simultaneously bars health care providers from providing abortion beyond 12 weeks of gestational age and "gender-altering procedures" for individuals younger than age 19. At once, this law targets women and other birthing people, transgender people, and transgender people capable of pregnancy. In Florida, 1 provision of Senate Bill 266 (2023) bars public institutions of higher education from offering "general education core courses" that "distort significant historical events or include a curriculum that teaches identity politics . . . or is based on theories that systemic racism, sexism, oppression, and privilege are inherent in the institutions of the United States." Another provision of the same law prohibits the use of state or federal funds for activities that "advocate for diversity, equity, and inclusion." As a whole, the statute targets multiple (and multiply) marginalized populations, including Black people and other people of color, LGBQ people, transgender people, women and people capable of pregnancy, and groups at the intersections of all of these categories—all of whom are priority populations for diversity, equity, and inclusion initiatives.

Third, discriminatory laws may impact individuals differently depending on their social positions. For example, a nationwide abortion ban would greatly increase pregnancy-related mortality, but the new harms would not be equitably distributed; instead, modeling predicts that additional deaths would be concentrated among non-Hispanic Black birthing people—those at the intersection of marginalized social positions because of gender and race—mirroring longstanding racial disparities in maternal mortality.[24] In these ways, discriminatory laws can disproportionately burden people who experience multiple sources of marginalization.

NEW WAVE(S) OF DISCRIMINATORY US LEGISLATION

Between January 1, 2020, and January 1, 2024, 30 US states enacted laws that adversely target 1 or more of the following groups: Black people and other people of color, LGBQ people, transgender people, and women and other people with the capacity for pregnancy (Table 1).

TABLE 1— Example State Laws That Target Marginalized Groups in the United States, Enacted January 1, 2020–January 1, 2024

State	Black People and Other People of Color	LGBQ People	Transgender People	Women and Other People With the Capacity for Pregnancy
Alabama	. . .	HB 322	SB 184	Ala Code §26-23H-4
Arizona	SB 2906	SB 1399	HB 1138	Ariz Rev Stat Ann §36-2326
Arkansas	SB 627	SB 294	HB 1156	Ark Code Ann §5-61-401 et seq.
Florida	HB 241	HB 1557	HB 1557	Fla Stat §390.0111
Georgia	HB 1084	SB 226	SB 140	Ga Code Ann §16-12-141
Idaho	HB 377	HB 190	HB 71	Idaho Code Ann §18-622
Indiana	HB 1447	HB 1608	HB 1041	Ind Code Ann §16-34-2-1
Iowa	HF 802	SF 496	HF 2416	SF 496
Kansas	. . .	. . .	HB 2238	HB 2184
Kentucky	SB 1	SB 150	SB 83	Ky Rev Stat Ann §311.722
Louisiana	. . .	SB 7	SB 44	La Rev Stat Ann §40:1061
Mississippi	SB 2113	SB 2346	HB 1125	Miss Code Ann §41-41-45
Missouri	SB 15	. . .	SB 49	Mo Rev Stat §188.017
Montana	. . .	HB 303	SB 99	HB 303
Nebraska	. . .	. . .	LB 574	LB 574
New Hampshire	HB 2	. . .	. . .	. . .
North Carolina	SL 2023-62	SL 2023-106	HB 808	NC Sess Laws 2023-14
North Dakota	HB 1508	HB 1111	HB 1254	SB 1250
Ohio	. . .	. . .	. . .	Ohio Rev Code Ann §2919.195(A)
Oklahoma	HB 1775	HB 3092	SB 615	Okla Stat tit 63, §1-731.4
Pennsylvania	. . .	. . .	. . .	HB 611
South Carolina	HB 4100	. . .	H4608	S 474
South Dakota	HB 1012	. . .	SB 46	SD Codified Laws §22-17-5.1
Tennessee	SB 623	. . .	HB 1895	SB 1257
Texas	HB 3979	HB 900	SB 14	Tex Health & Safety Code Ann §170A.001 et seq.
Utah	SB 55	SB 55	HB 11	Utah Code Ann §76-7a-201
Virginia	HB 127	. . .	. . .	. . .
West Virginia	. . .	. . .	HB 2007	W Va Code §16-2R-3
Wisconsin	. . .	. . .	. . .	Wis Stat §940.04
Wyoming	. . .	. . .	SF 133	HB 152

Note. HB = House Bill; HF = House File; LB = Legislative Bill; LGBQ = lesbian, gay, bisexual, or queer; S = Senate General Bill; SB = Senate Bill; SF = Senate File. Data were compiled across publicly available legislative trackers that monitor laws affecting Black people and other people of color (https://crtforward.law.ucla.edu, https://datavisualizations.heritage.org/education/critical-race-theory-legislation-tracker, https://citizensrenewingamerica.com/issues/state-tracker-crt-legislation), LGBQ people (https://www.aclu.org/legislative-attacks-on-lgbtq-rights, https://www.lgbtmap.org/equality-maps, https://www.equalityfederation.org/state-legislation), transgender people (https://translegislation.com, https://www.tracktranslegislation.com, https://www.hrc.org/resources/attacks-on-gender-affirming-care-by-state-map, https://www.equalityfederation.org/tracker/cumulative-anti-transgender), and women and other people capable of pregnancy (https://reproductiverights.org/maps/abortion-laws-by-state, https://www.nytimes.com/interactive/2022/us/abortion-laws-roe-v-wade.html, https://www.guttmacher.org/state-legislation-tracker, https://www.kff.org/womens-health-policy/report/state-and-federal-reproductive-rights-and-abortion-litigation-tracker). The table shows trackers' classifications without modification.

Twenty-five of these states passed laws targeting more than 1 stigmatized group. We selected these 4 marginalized groups as illustrative for our analysis, although similar efforts could, and should, illuminate laws affecting additional marginalized populations, such as immigrants, incarcerated individuals, people with disabilities, and people living in poverty. We do not focus on the causes of law, but we note that this time encompasses important political shifts, including a new presidential administration, increased polarization in state legislatures, and changes in the composition of federal courts that evaluate the constitutionality of state laws.

Our synthesis includes laws that were passed by the state legislature and signed by the governor or that had a governor's veto overridden. We include "trigger" laws that took effect after the Supreme Court's decision in *Dobbs v Jackson Women's Health Organization*, laws that pre-empted localities from passing protective ordinances, and laws that were enacted but struck down by courts or reversed. We adopt the classifications applied by legislation trackers, which use varying methodologies. For example, some but not all trackers include laws that are facially neutral but susceptible to discriminatory application (e.g., laws that allow religious objections to adoption placements can be used to discriminate against LGBQ couples). Some laws are specific to health care practice (e.g., restrictions on gender-affirming care), while others focus on other domains (e.g., laws that bar schools from enforcing the use of students' preferred pronouns). Our tables are therefore illustrative rather than comprehensive, and Table 1 includes the trackers we used and an example citation for each category of law. Where any tracker classified a law as discriminatory to a group of interest, we included it. Relying on publicly available trackers has inherent limitations. They can be simultaneously underinclusive (i.e., failing to find or classify relevant laws) and overinclusive (i.e., including laws with a vague or attenuated relationship to the populations of interest). Strengths, however, are that this method saves resources, making it feasible to monitor multiple types of law simultaneously; public trackers are accessible and therefore drive advocacy, practice, and conversations about law; and our model of expressive impacts involves public perceptions of law, for which public trackers are instructive.

From an intersectional perspective, the most common pattern was for states to pass legislation targeting every 1 of the 4 groups of interest (either separately or in the same statute), which occurred in 14 states. The next most common patterns occurred in states that passed laws targeting transgender people and women (4 states); laws targeting Black people and other people of color, transgender people, and women and other people capable of pregnancy (4 states); and laws targeting LGBQ people, transgender people, and women and other people capable of pregnancy (3 states). Three states passed legislation targeting women and other people capable of pregnancy but were not identified as targeting other groups; 2 states passed legislation targeting Black people and other people of color but not other groups. Sixteen of the 30 states passed at least 1 law that simultaneously targeted more than 1 of the 4 identified groups in the same bill or statute (Table 2).

These patterns identify how recent discriminatory legislation has proceeded simultaneously on multiple fronts, and how lawmaking acts to burden the same groups repeatedly across jurisdictions. Where a state has recently passed laws discriminating against transgender individuals, laws burdening women and other birthing people are also likely in that state. And where one state legislature passes a new law burdening LGBQ people, other states may follow. Across states, we note that populations at the intersections of the chosen marginalized groups, such as LGBQ people of color or transgender people capable of pregnancy, are repeatedly exposed to the unique and synergistic consequences of these laws.

A CALL FOR ACTION THROUGH PRACTICE AND RESEARCH

Across many US states, discriminatory legislation is rolling back dignity, opportunities, and material resources for marginalized groups. We have illustrated this point with reference to 4 marginalized populations, although additional analyses could and should include many other groups (e.g., incarcerated people, disabled people, immigrants). Drawing on extensive previous work in legal epidemiology, the health consequences of stigma, and intersectionality, we predict that exposure to discriminatory legislation is likely to produce deleterious health outcomes for marginalized group members.[12] We therefore view this constellation of laws as a concerted force that threatens the health of multiple marginalized groups. Because more than half of US people experience 1 or more sources of marginalization, there is an urgent need for a coordinated, multilateral effort that counters these laws and addresses their likely health consequences. Legislators, legislative staff, advocacy groups, and political processes are integral to this response, but health care clinicians, institutions, and researchers also have a critical role to play. Indeed, intersectionality praxis, which Bowleg has labeled the "fourth wave" of intersectionality within public health, compels health care clinicians, institutions, and researchers to act.[20]

Much of health care research and practice focuses on 1 population or issue at a time. Where discriminatory laws affect specific groups or legal questions, targeted responses are essential. Marginalized populations have differences in social, economic, and political exclusion; historical context; care needs; and structural health risks,

TABLE 2— **Example State Laws That Simultaneously Target Multiple Marginalized Groups in the United States, Enacted January 1, 2020–January 1, 2024**

State	Law	Year	Black People and Other People of Color	LGBQ People	Transgender People	Women and Other People Capable of Pregnancy
Alabama	HB 322	2022		X	X	
Arizona	HB 2161	2022	X	X	X	X
Arizona	SB 1399	2022		X	X	X
Arizona	HB 2439	2022	X	X	X	
Arkansas	SB 294	2023	X	X	X	X
Arkansas	HB 1615	2023		X	X	
Florida	HB 1069	2023	X	X	X	X
Florida	SB 266	2023	X	X	X	X
Florida	SB 1382	2023	X	X	X	
Florida	S 1580	2023		X	X	X
Florida	HB 7	2022	X	X	X	
Florida	HB 1557	2022		X	X	X
Georgia	SB 226	2023		X	X	X
Indiana	HB 1608	2023		X	X	
Iowa	SF 496	2023	X	X	X	X
Kentucky	SB 150	2023		X	X	
Louisiana	SB 7	2023		X	X	
Louisiana	HB 61	2023		X	X	
Louisiana	HB 77	2023		X	X	
Louisiana	SB 162	2023		X	X	
Mississippi	SB 2346	2023		X	X	
Montana	HB 303	2023		X	X	X
Nebraska	LB 574	2023			X	X
North Carolina	SL 2023-106	2023		X	X	
North Dakota	HB 1205	2023		X	X	X
North Dakota	HB 1111	2023		X	X	X
Oklahoma	SB 404	2023		X	X	
Oklahoma	HB 3092	2022	X	X	X	X
Texas	HB 900	2023		X	X	
Utah	SB 97	2023		X	X	
Utah	SB 55	2022	X	X	X	X

Note. HB = House Bill; LB = Legislative Bill; LGBQ = lesbian, gay, bisexual, or queer; S = Senate General Bill; SB = Senate Bill; SF = Senate File; SL = Session Laws. Data were compiled across publicly available legislative trackers that monitor laws affecting Black people and other people of color (https://crtforward.law.ucla.edu, https://datavisualizations.heritage.org/education/critical-race-theory-legislation-tracker, https://citizensrenewingamerica.com/issues/state-tracker-crt-legislation), LGBQ people (https://www.aclu.org/legislative-attacks-on-lgbtq-rights, https://www.lgbtmap.org/equality-maps, https://www.equalityfederation.org/state-legislation), transgender people (https://translegislation.com, https://www.tracktranslegislation.com, https://www.hrc.org/resources/attacks-on-gender-affirming-care-by-state-map, https://www.equalityfederation.org/tracker/cumulative-anti-transgender), and women and other people capable of pregnancy (https://reproductiverights.org/maps/abortion-laws-by-state, https://www.nytimes.com/interactive/2022/us/abortion-laws-roe-v-wade.html, https://www.guttmacher.org/state-legislation-tracker, https://www.kff.org/womens-health-policy/report/state-and-federal-reproductive-rights-and-abortion-litigation-tracker). The table shows trackers' classifications without modification.

and they have diverse pathways toward equity and justice. Health care stakeholders have also foregrounded laws that directly restrict health care practice, such as laws that penalize providers of abortion or gender-affirming care.

Although particularized responses to laws that burden specific populations and clinical services are imperative, relying solely on a compartmentalized response also has drawbacks. An issue-by-issue view can overlook the acute damage that laws can do to people who simultaneously hold more than 1 marginalized social position. Indeed, systematic reviews now identify hundreds of studies documenting differential health burdens (e.g., chronic conditions, sexually transmitted infections, suicidal ideation, substance use) among people who experience multiple forms of social marginalization.[21,22] Moreover, these seemingly distinct discriminatory laws co-occur in ways that shift power and opportunity away from multiple marginalized groups simultaneously. Viewing specific populations or issues in isolation can obscure how multiple laws work together to shape environment, behavior, and health outcomes. A wider, intersectional lens can capture opportunities for collaboration, harnessing the much-needed power and strength of groups experiencing a common set of legislative threats. Indeed, intersectionality, Bowleg notes, "is fundamentally a resistance project" that demands action,[20(p89)] such as efforts to mitigate legislative threats, to work with policymakers to reshape existing laws, and to prevent the passage of harmful new laws. These movements should also recognize and defer to leaders, advocacy efforts, expertise, and priorities from within multiply marginalized groups.

The skills and political capital of clinicians and institutions can be formidable forces in the response to discriminatory laws. First, clinicians in every specialty have patients experiencing the burdens of these laws, whether they be direct (e.g., inability to access gender-affirming care) or indirect (e.g., increased discrimination attributable to not being able to use a gender-congruent bathroom). Clinicians should therefore prepare to identify and treat potential increases in psychological and physical harms among marginalized patients. Second, health care institutions and clinicians can develop practice norms that resist multiple forms of discrimination. These include promoting structural competency[25]; providing staff and provider training in equity-oriented, person-centered care that addresses historical and contemporary discrimination[26,27]; hiring, supporting, and retaining providers and staff from marginalized communities; and enforcing hospital and clinic policies that support equitable treatment and accountability. We note that many health care providers are navigating an unprecedented and uncertain landscape of sanctions, including criminal penalties, licensing consequences, or fines for providing certain forms of care (e.g., abortion, gender-affirming care); providers will need to decide the best-available course of action depending on where they practice.

Third, health care institutions and clinicians—particularly in privately organized health care systems, as is common in the United States—wield expertise, influence, and material resources, which generate political capital. Given the health consequences that are likely to follow discriminatory legislation, health care institutions and clinicians can use their political influence to oppose not only laws restricting medical practice but also discriminatory legislation in other areas (e.g., laws banning transgender students from school athletics). Because discriminatory legislation is likely to exacerbate health inequities among marginalized groups, clinicians and health care institutions have a professional interest in opposing these damaging laws.

Health research on state laws can also be more powerful when it recognizes how laws intersect, including how this intersection impacts subgroups facing multiple forms of discrimination simultaneously. Legal epidemiological methods should be used to track and systematically map discriminatory laws that are likely to impact population health and should focus on linkages between these laws and health outcomes.[28] Furthermore, researchers should collect demographic information that allows the identification of diverse subgroups, the study of multiple laws, and the ways that laws' compliance and expressive functions influence environment, behavior, and health. Research funders can support this work by prioritizing projects that consider the interplay among state laws, stigma, and health among marginalized groups.

Discriminatory laws undermine the autonomy and health of marginalized people, to the advantage of dominant social groups. A coordinated threat demands a collective and intersectional response, and the clinicians, institutions, and researchers that care for marginalized patients have compelling reasons to join this work. AJPH

ABOUT THE AUTHORS

Kristen Underhill is with Cornell Law School, Ithaca, NY, and the Department of Population Health Sciences, Weill Cornell Medical College, New York, NY. Valerie A. Earnshaw is with the Department of Human Development and Family Sciences, University of Delaware, Newark. Kimberly M. Nelson is with the Department of Community Health Sciences, Boston University School of Public Health, and the Department of Psychiatry, Chobanian & Avedisian School of Medicine, Boston University, Boston, MA.

CORRESPONDENCE

Correspondence should be sent to Kimberly Nelson, PhD, MPH, Boston University School of Public Health, 801 Massachusetts Ave, 4th Floor, Boston, MA 02118 (e-mail: knel@bu.edu). Reprints can be ordered at https://www.ajph.org by clicking the "Reprints" link.

PUBLICATION INFORMATION

Full Citation: Underhill K, Earnshaw VA, Nelson KM. The synergistic health threats of state laws targeting marginalized groups in the United States. *Am J Public Health*. 2024;114(12):1335–1343.

Acceptance Date: July 25, 2024.

DOI: https://doi.org/10.2105/AJPH.2024.307830

ORCID iDs:

Valerie A. Earnshaw https://orcid.org/0000-0002-4147-3301

Kimberly M. Nelson https://orcid.org/0000-0001-8893-5764

CONTRIBUTORS

K. Underhill and K. Nelson conceptualized the essay. K. Underhill led the legal analysis. K. Nelson acquired the funding. K. Underhill and K. Nelson drafted the article with extensive input from V. Earnshaw. All authors reviewed and edited the article.

ACKNOWLEDGMENTS

This work is supported by the National Institutes of Mental Health (R01MH119892, Principal Investigator: Nelson).

We are grateful to Hannah Knapp-Broas for assistance compiling data from public legislation trackers.

Note. The content of this publication is solely the responsibility of the authors and does not represent the official views of the National Institutes of Health. The National Institutes of Health had no role in the design and conduct of the study; collection, management, analysis, and interpretation of the data; preparation, review, or approval of the manuscript; or decision to submit the manuscript for publication.

CONFLICTS OF INTEREST

The authors have no conflicts to report.

HUMAN PARTICIPANT PROTECTION

Human participant protection was not required because this work did not involve human participants.

REFERENCES

1. Burris S, Wagenaar AC, Swanson J, Ibrahim JK, Wood J, Mello MM. Making the case for laws that improve health: a framework for public health law research. *Milbank Q*. 2010;88(2):169–210. https://doi.org/10.1111/j.1468-0009.2010.00595.x
2. Burris S, Berman ML, Penn M, Holiday TR. *The New Public Health Law: A Transdisciplinary Approach to Practice and Advocacy*. New York, NY: Oxford University Press; 2022. https://doi.org/10.1093/oso/9780197615973.001.0001
3. Gonzales G, Ehrenfeld JM. The association between state policy environments and self-rated health disparities for sexual minorities in the United States. *Int J Environ Res Public Health*. 2018;15(6):1136. https://doi.org/10.3390/ijerph15061136
4. Rapp KS, Volpe VV, Hale TL, Quartararo DF. State-level sexism and gender disparities in health care access and quality in the United States. *J Health Soc Behav*. 2022;63(1):2–18. https://doi.org/10.1177/00221465211058153
5. Jahn JL, Zubizarreta D, Chen JT, et al. Legislating inequity: structural racism in groups of state laws and associations with premature mortality rates: study examines the combined harmful effects of state laws and structural racism's association with premature mortality rates. *Health Aff (Millwood)*. 2023;42(10):1325–1333. https://doi.org/10.1377/hlthaff.2023.00471
6. Bowleg L. The problem with the phrase *women and minorities:* intersectionality—an important theoretical framework for public health. *Am J Public Health*. 2012;102(7):1267–1273. https://doi.org/10.2105/AJPH.2012.300750
7. Gostin LO, Monahan JT, Kaldor J, et al. The legal determinants of health: harnessing the power of law for global health and sustainable development. *Lancet*. 2019;393(10183):1857–1910. https://doi.org/10.1016/S0140-6736(19)30233-8
8. Hatzenbuehler ML, Lattanner MR, McKetta S, Pachankis JE. Structural stigma and LGBTQ+ health: a narrative review of quantitative studies [erratum in *Lancet Public Health*. 2024;9(4):e217]. *Lancet Public Health*. 2024;9(2):e109–e127. https://doi.org/10.1016/S2468-2667(23)00312-2
9. Wang E, Clymer J, Davis-Hayes C, Buttenheim A. Nonmedical exemptions from school immunization requirements: a systematic review. *Am J Public Health*. 2014;104(11):e62–e84. https://doi.org/10.2105/AJPH.2014.302190
10. Slavova S, Rock P, Bush HM, Quesinberry D, Walsh SL. Signal of increased opioid overdose during COVID-19 from emergency medical services data. *Drug Alcohol Depend*. 2020;214:108176. https://doi.org/10.1016/j.drugalcdep.2020.108176
11. Burris S. Stigma and the law. *Lancet*. 2006;367(9509):529–531. https://doi.org/10.1016/S0140-6736(06)68185-3
12. Hatzenbuehler ML, Phelan JC, Link BG. Stigma as a fundamental cause of population health inequalities. *Am J Public Health*. 2013;103(5):813–821. https://doi.org/10.2105/AJPH.2012.301069
13. Link BG, Phelan JC. Conceptualizing stigma. *Annu Rev Sociol*. 2001;27(1):363–385. https://doi.org/10.1146/annurev.soc.27.1.363
14. Lopez G. Women are getting harassed in bathrooms because of anti-transgender hysteria. *Vox*. May 19, 2016. Available at: https://www.vox.com/2016/5/18/11690234/women-bathrooms-harassment. Accessed June 27, 2024.
15. Polgreen L. Ron DeSantis knows that the best place to humiliate people is in the bathroom. *New York Times*. May 19, 2023. Available at: https://www.nytimes.com/2023/05/19/opinion/anti-trans-bathroom-laws-florida.html. Accessed June 27, 2024.
16. Atwood S, Morgenroth T, Olson KR. Gender essentialism and benevolent sexism in anti-trans rhetoric. *Soc Issues Policy Rev*. 2024;18(1):171–193. https://doi.org/10.1111/sipr.12099
17. Krieger N. Measures of racism, sexism, heterosexism, and gender binarism for health equity research: from structural injustice to embodied harm—an ecosocial analysis. *Annu Rev Public Health*. 2020;41(1):37–62. https://doi.org/10.1146/annurev-publhealth-040119-094017
18. Caughey D, Warshaw C. The dynamics of state policy liberalism, 1936–2014. *Am J Pol Sci*. 2016;60(4):899–913. https://doi.org/10.1111/ajps.12219
19. Crenshaw K. Demarginalizing the intersection of race and sex: a Black feminist critique of antidiscrimination doctrine, feminist theory and antiracist politics. *Univ Chic Leg Forum*. 1989;1989(1):139–167.
20. Bowleg L. Evolving intersectionality within public health: from analysis to action. *Am J Public Health*. 2021;111(1):88–90. https://doi.org/10.2105/AJPH.2020.306031
21. Bauer GR, Churchill SM, Mahendran M, Walwyn C, Lizotte D, Villa-Rueda AA. Intersectionality in quantitative research: a systematic review of its emergence and applications of theory and methods. *SSM Popul Health*. 2021;14:100798. https://doi.org/10.1016/j.ssmph.2021.100798
22. Harari L, Lee C. Intersectionality in quantitative health disparities research: a systematic review of challenges and limitations in empirical studies. *Soc Sci Med*. 2021;277:113876. https://doi.org/10.1016/j.socscimed.2021.113876
23. Denise EJ. Multiple disadvantaged statuses and health: the role of multiple forms of discrimination. *J Health Soc Behav*. 2014;55(1):3–19. https://doi.org/10.1177/0022146514521215
24. Stevenson AJ. The pregnancy-related mortality impact of a total abortion ban in the United States: a research note on increased deaths due to remaining pregnant. *Demography*. 2021;58(6):2019–2028. https://doi.org/10.1215/00703370-9585908
25. Metzl JM, Hansen H. Structural competency: theorizing a new medical engagement with stigma and inequality. *Soc Sci Med*. 2014;103:126–133. https://doi.org/10.1016/j.socscimed.2013.06.032
26. Håkansson Eklund J, Holmström IK, Kumlin T, et al. "Same same or different?" A review of reviews of person-centered and patient-centered care. *Patient Educ Couns*. 2019;102(1):3–11. https://doi.org/10.1016/j.pec.2018.08.029
27. Green TL, Zapata JY, Brown HW, Hagiwara N. Rethinking bias to achieve maternal health equity: changing organizations, not just individuals. *Obstet Gynecol*. 2021;137(5):935–940. https://doi.org/10.1097/AOG.0000000000004363
28. Burris S, Hitchcock L, Ibrahim J, Penn M, Ramanathan T. Policy surveillance: a vital public health practice comes of age. *J Health Polit Policy Law*. 2016;41(6):1151–1173. https://doi.org/10.1215/03616878-3665931

An Inventory of Proposed and Enacted Sugar-Sweetened Beverage Policies at the State, Local, and Tribal Levels in the United States, 2014–2023

Jennie N. Davis, PhD, RDN, Shatabdi Goon, MSc, Jessie Gouck, MUP, Sarah E. Solar, BS, Sally Mancini, MPH, Alberto M. Ortega Hinojosa, PhD, MPH, James Krieger, MD, MPH, and Jennifer Falbe, ScD, MPH

See also State Laws Targeting Marginalized Groups, pp. 1322–1364.

Objectives. To inventory and describe trends in proposal and enactment of US sugar-sweetened beverage (SSB) policies at state, local, and Tribal levels, 2014–2023.

Methods. We systematically searched 6 policy databases in 2021 (updated May 2023) using SSB-related search terms, identifying additional policies through snowball and online searches and a survey of food-policy experts. We reviewed 10 821 policies for inclusion and quantitatively coded included policies.

Results. The inventory included 400 (321 unique [i.e., excluding companion]) policies meeting criteria: 335 (256 unique) state-, 63 local-, and 2 Tribal-level policies. From 2014 to 2023, 11% of unique state-, 92% of local-, and 100% of Tribal-level proposed policies were enacted. Across jurisdictions, the most frequently proposed policies related to excise taxes, restaurant children's meals, nutrition standards, and the Supplemental Nutrition Assistance Program, while the largest proportions of enacted policies related to restaurant children's meals, nutrition standards, education, and procurement. More policies were proposed and enacted in California and New York than other states, and in 2017 (proposed) and 2016 (enacted).

Conclusions. This comprehensive inventory of US SSB policies provides information to inform future SSB policy development and diffusion. (*Am J Public Health*. 2024;114(12):1344–1353. https://doi.org/10.2105/AJPH.2024.307855)

AJPH December 2024, Vol. 114, No. 12

Reducing sugar-sweetened beverage (SSB) consumption is a public health priority.[1,2] SSBs are the leading source of dietary added sugars[3] and increase the risk of cardiometabolic and dental diseases.[4,5] Policies are an important tool for reducing SSB marketing, availability, sales, and consumption. Policies like SSB excise taxes are recommended by public health organizations, such as the American Heart Association and World Health Organization.[1,2] SSB policies in the United States and abroad have reduced SSB purchases and consumption,[6,7] and multicomponent policy approaches are recommended to maximize reach and effectiveness (i.e., a policy requiring both SSB warning labels and restricting SSB advertising to children, as in Chile).[8,9] Excise tax policies, which are expected to reduce health care spending, are especially cost-effective,[10] and in the United States, revenue generated from SSB taxes has supported health and equity programs (e.g., universal prekindergarten, safe drinking water availability).[11,12]

Despite the utility of policy for addressing SSB consumption, there is a lack of research identifying and characterizing SSB-related policies. Previous studies have described policies in other areas (e.g., cardiometabolic health, portion sizes, ultraprocessed foods, and food service guidelines[13,14]) or a subset of SSB-related policies (e.g., warning labels).[15,16] However, no comprehensive inventory of SSB policies exists. An inventory of proposed and enacted SSB-related policies could (1) serve as a resource to jurisdictions designing policies to meet their specific needs, (2) provide researchers with an understanding of the SSB policy landscape to facilitate evaluation of existing policies and stimulate the development and testing of novel policies, and (3) provide information for policymakers, practitioners, and advocates contemplating or actively seeking adoption of SSB policies. Therefore, our objective was to identify, inventory, and summarize high-level characteristics of proposed and enacted SSB policies at local, state, and Tribal levels in the United States from 2014 to May of 2023, and describe trends in proposal and enactment. We excluded the federal level because SSB policy activities have been concentrated at state and local levels.

METHODS

We searched for local- (city or county), state- (including Washington, DC), and Tribal-level policies, bills, resolutions, and ordinances and municipal codes (hereafter: "policies") that were proposed or enacted and explicitly addressed reducing SSB consumption or availability (e.g., tax, advertising, warning label policies) or that indirectly addressed SSB consumption (e.g., by focusing on added sugars). Policies reintroduced in a new legislative session were counted as separate "unique policies." State-level bicameral policies (companion bills in both legislative bodies) were individually coded but considered a single unique policy in analyses describing focus areas and trends. We limited our search to US policies proposed or enacted January 1, 2014, through May 31, 2023. January 1, 2014, was selected to coincide with the enactment year of the first SSB excise tax in Berkeley, California,[15] and the Healthy Diné Nation Act, which established a 2% sales tax on "minimal-to-no-nutritional-value" foods and beverages, including SSBs.[17]

We excluded policies not directly applicable to our objective:

1. federal policies, US territory, or non-US policies;
2. institutional (e.g., hospitals, universities) "policies" or guidelines not enacted by government;
3. school nutrition standards policies (e.g., National School Breakfast or Lunch Programs, school wellness policies [excluded because of extensive existing research[18–20]]);
4. policies related only to increasing drinking water access without mentioning reducing SSB availability or consumption;
5. beverage tax policies without a main focus on sweetened beverages (e.g., taxing all beverages, bottle deposit fee);
6. policies intended to repeal, oppose, or preempt SSB policies (e.g., California's local SSB tax preemption);
7. "skeleton" policies (policies submitted in outline form with the intention to add specific language later); and
8. policies otherwise not relevant. Appendix A, Table A (available as a supplement to the online version of this article at https://ajph.org) provides examples of excluded policies.

Databases and Search Strategy

We conducted systematic searches, using predefined search terms related to SSBs, in 6 databases (Appendix A, Table B): American Legal Publishing Code Library (American Legal Publishing Code Library, Cincinnati, OH), Ballotpedia (Lucy Burns Institute, Middleton, WI), Healthy Food Policy Project (Center for Agriculture and Food Systems at Vermont Law School, Royalton, VT), Municode Code Library (CivicPlus, Manhattan, KS), Nexis Uni (LexisNexis, New York, NY), and Westlaw (Thomson Reuters, Toronto, Canada). Manual searches of relevant Web sites, "snowball" searches (identifying policies in publication reference lists), and policies known by the research team were also included. Following removal of duplicates, 4815 local, state, and Tribal policies were independently screened for relevance by 2 coauthors (J. N. D. and S. G.), with uncertainties resolved through discussion (Appendix A, Figure A). We conducted initial searches in June 2021; we conducted updated searches in American Legal Publishing Code Library, Ballotpedia, Healthy Food Policy Project, Municode, Nexis Uni, and Westlaw databases in May 2023 to identify additional policies since June 2021.

Local and Tribal Policy Survey

To identify local and Tribal policies missed by our searches because of the lack of comprehensive local and Tribal policy databases, we purposively surveyed organizations known to the study team to have expertise in local or Tribal food policy: 5 nongovernmental organizations and 4 university centers (3 with Tribal policy expertise). From June through September 2023, 8 individuals in 6 organizations completed the survey: 2 university centers with Tribal policy expertise and 3 national nongovernmental organizations and 1 university center focused on food policy generally. The survey (Supplemental Material in Appendix A) provided participants with a list of identified local- and Tribal-level policies and asked them to identify any additional policies. Of 19 policies submitted, 8 nonduplicate relevant policies were added to the sample (Appendix A, Figure A).

Data Coding and Analysis

Key policy characteristics coded were policy focus area(s), jurisdictional level (local [i.e., city or county], state, Tribal territory), reference number (e.g., SB 123), policy title, year introduced, year enacted (if applicable), current status (e.g., proposed only or enacted), companion policy if relevant, and a Web link to the policy. In June 2024, we checked for status updates of local policies proposed since 2021 because consideration of local policies is not limited to a single legislation session. The 14 non–mutually exclusive SSB policy focus areas (Appendix A, Table C) were

1. education and outreach,
2. excise tax,
3. healthy checkout,
4. healthy procurement,
5. healthy retail,
6. marketing and advertising,
7. nutrition standards (subfocus areas: before- and after-school programs, child care, day camps, healthy meetings, hospitals, vending machines on state, city, or county property),
8. portion size,
9. research and evaluation,
10. restaurant children's meals,
11. sales tax,
12. Supplemental Nutrition Assistance Program (SNAP),
13. warning labels, and
14. water.

We coded a single policy with multiple focus areas (e.g., excise tax and warning labels) for each focus area, with the primary focus area being the one listed first in the policy. Likewise, we coded secondary, tertiary, etc., focus areas based on the next subsequent area listed. Policy characteristics were coded by one coauthor (J. N. D.) and verified by a second coauthor (S. G.). We coded proposed, enacted, and companion policies. If there were multiple versions of a policy within a single session (e.g., amendments), we coded the last version.

Analyses were descriptive, including policy frequency and percentage enacted by jurisdictional level, focus area, state, and year. In analyses describing the frequency of policy focus areas, a single policy with multiple focus areas contributed to each focus area. A policy that was reintroduced in a new legislative session was counted as a separate, unique policy. In analyses of policy frequency by year, the policy year was the year each policy was introduced for proposed-only policies. For enacted policies, the policy year was the year of enactment; the reason we used enactment year is because, for all state policies, the enactment year is the same as the year introduced, and for local enacted policies with retrievable data on year introduced (36%), 71% had the same introduction and enactment year. We conducted coding in Excel (version 2306, Microsoft Corporation, Redmond, WA), analysis with Stata (version 18, StataCorp College Station, TX), and mapping with Tableau (version 2023.3, Salesforce, San Francisco, CA).

RESULTS

In total, we included 400 proposed SSB policies (including companion) between January 1, 2014, and May 31, 2023, in the inventory: 63 local-, 335 state-, and 2 Tribal-level policies. The 335 state-level proposed policies included 79 companion policies. After excluding companion policies, there were 256 unique state-level proposed policies, for a total of 321 unique local, state, and Tribal proposed policies. At the local level, 58 (92%) of the 63 proposed policies were enacted versus 28 (11%) of the 256 state-level proposed policies. The 2 Tribal policies were enacted. Hereafter, we present results by unique policy only (i.e., companion policies are described as 1 unique policy). Characteristics of all policies (e.g., focus area, status) and their Web links are included in Appendix B (available as a supplement to the online version of this article at https://ajph.org).

Policy Focus Area

Figure 1 shows the frequency of unique proposed policies in each focus area overall by jurisdictional level and status. Across all levels of proposed policies (n = 321), the 5 most frequent focus areas were excise taxes (n = 80; 25% of proposed policies), restaurant children's meals (n = 79; 25%), nutrition standards (n = 48; 15%), SNAP (n = 29; 9%), and warning labels (n = 28; 9%). Of the 88 enacted policies across levels, the 5 most frequently enacted focus areas were restaurant children's meals (n = 31; 35%), nutrition standards (n = 27; 31%), education and outreach (n = 12; 14%), healthy procurement (n = 11; 13%), and excise taxes (n = 7; 8%). Across levels, focus areas with the highest probability of enactment were healthy retail (100% of only 2 proposed policies), education and outreach (92% of 13), healthy checkout (67% of 3), nutrition standards (56% of 48), and healthy procurement (46% of 24). The focus areas least likely to be enacted

	All Levels			State			Local			Tribal		
	Total Proposed, no. (%[b])	Enacted, no. (%[b])	Percent Enacted, %[c]	Total Proposed, no. (%[b])	Enacted, no. (%[b])	Percent Enacted, %[c]	Total Proposed, no. (%[b])	Enacted, no. (%[b])	Percent Enacted, %[c]	Total Proposed, no. (%[b])	Enacted, no. (%[b])	Percent Enacted, %[c]
Total SSB policies[a]	321 (100)	88 (100)	27	256 (100)	28 (100)	11	63 (100)	58 (100)	92	2 (100)	2 (100)	100
Policies[a] by focus area[b]												
Education and outreach	13 (4)	12 (14)	92	13 (5)	12 (43)	92	0 (0)	0 (0)	...	0 (0)	0 (0)	...
Excise tax	80 (25)	7 (8)	9	70 (27)	0 (0)	0	10 (16)	7 (12)	70	0 (0)	0 (0)	...
Healthy checkout	3 (1)	2 (2)	67	1 (0.4)	0 (0)	0	2 (3)	2 (3)	100	0 (0)	0 (0)	...
Healthy procurement	24 (7)	11 (13)	46	14 (5)	1 (4)	7	9 (14)	9 (16)	100	1 (50)	1 (50)	100
Healthy retail	2 (1)	2 (2)	100	0 (0)	0 (0)	...	2 (3)	2 (3)	100	0 (0)	0 (0)	...
Marketing and advertising	15 (5)	1 (1)	7	15 (6)	1 (4)	7	0 (0)	0 (0)	...	0 (0)	0 (0)	...
Nutrition standards total	48 (15)	27 (31)	56	26 (10)	5 (18)	19	21 (33)	21 (36)	100	1 (50)	1 (50)	100
Before/ after school	7 (2)	1 (1)	14	7 (3)	1 (4)	14	0 (0)	0 (0)	...	0 (0)	0 (0)	...
Childcare	9 (3)	3 (3)	33	8 (3)	2 (7)	25	1 (2)	1 (2)	100	0 (0)	0 (0)	...
Children's day camps	1 (0.3)	1 (1)	100	0 (0)	0 (0)	...	1 (2)	1 (2)	100	0 (0)	0 (0)	...
Healthy meetings	5 (2)	5 (6)	100	1 (0.4)	1 (4)	100	4 (6)	4 (7)	100	0 (0)	0 (0)	...
Vending on public property	26 (8)	17 (19)	65	10 (4)	1 (4)	10	15 (24)	15 (26)	100	1 (50)	1 (50)	100
Portion size	3 (1)	0 (0)	0	3 (1)	0 (0)	0	0 (0)	0 (0)	...	0 (0)	0 (0)	...
Research and evaluation	9 (3)	2 (2)	22	9 (4)	2 (7)	22	0 (0)	0 (0)	...	0 (0)	0 (0)	...
Restaurant children's meals	79 (25)	31 (35)	39	52 (20)	5 (18)	10	26 (41)	26 (45)	100	0 (0)	0 (0)	...
Sales tax	16 (5)	3 (3)	19	13 (5)	1 (4)	8	2 (3)	1 (2)	50	1 (50)	1 (50)	100
SNAP	29 (9)	0 (0)	0	29 (11)	0 (0)	0	0 (0)	0 (0)	...	0 (0)	0 (0)	...
Warning labels	28 (9)	3 (3)	11	24 (9)	0 (0)	0	4 (6)	3 (5)	75	0 (0)	0 (0)	...
Water	12 (4)	2 (2)	17	12 (5)	2 (7)	17	0 (0)	0 (0)	...	0 (0)	0 (0)	...

FIGURE 1— Frequency of Proposed and Enacted Unique Sugar-Sweetened Beverage Policies at the State, Local, and Tribal Levels: United States, 2014–2023

Note. SNAP = Supplemental Nutrition Assistance Program; SSB = sugar-sweetened beverage. Heat map shading was done separately by column. Darker shading indicates higher percentages within each column.

[a]The figure contains all unique policies, meaning that bicameral legislation (same policies introduced in both legislative bodies in the same session) were counted as 1 "unique" policy. "Proposed" indicates all policies that were proposed; "enacted" indicates all policies that were enacted and includes 3 local-level policies that were enacted and then repealed (2015, Davis, CA, Ordinance 2451 restaurant children's meals policy; 2017 Cook County, IL, Ordinance 16-5931 sales tax policy; 2016 San Francisco, CA, Article 42 warning label policy).

[b]Because focus areas are not mutually exclusive (i.e., 26 policies had multiple focus areas), the denominator for percentages of total proposed and enacted policies is the total number of total proposed or enacted SSB policies in the first row.

[c]Percentage of the total number of proposed policies that were enacted.

were SNAP (0% of 29 proposed policies), portion size (0% of 3), marketing and advertising (7% of 15), excise taxes (9% of 80), and warning labels (11% of 28). Of the enacted nutrition standards policies, 17 (65%) were for beverages sold in vending machines on public property. Twenty-six proposed policies (16 state, 9 local, 1 Tribal) had 2 or more focus areas; of these, 11 (44%) were enacted, 9 of which were local-level policies (Appendix B).

At the state level among all proposed policies (n = 256), the 5 most frequent focus areas were excise taxes (n = 70; 27%), restaurant children's meals (n = 52; 20%), SNAP (n = 29; 11%), nutrition standards (n = 26; 10%), and warning labels (n = 24; 9%). Among state enacted policies (n = 28), the 5 most frequent focus areas were education and outreach policies, which made up the bulk of enacted policies (n = 12; 43%), followed by nutrition standards (n = 5; 18%), restaurant children's meals (n = 5; 18%), research and evaluation (n = 2; 7%), and water (n = 2; 7%). State education and outreach policies had the highest probability of enactment (92% of 13 policies), followed by research and evaluation (22% of 9), nutrition standards (19% of 26), water (17% of 12), and restaurant children's meals (10% of 52). State-level excise tax, healthy checkout, portion size, SNAP, and warning labels had 0% probability of enactment.

Among local-level proposed policies (n = 63), the 5 most frequent focus areas were restaurant children's meals (n = 26; 41%), nutrition standards (n = 21; 33%), excise taxes (n = 10; 16%), healthy procurement (n = 9; 14%), and warning labels (n = 4; 6%). Among local enacted policies (n = 58), the 5 most frequent focus areas were restaurant children's meals (n = 26; 45%), nutrition standards (n = 21; 36%), healthy procurement (n = 9; 16%), excise taxes (n = 7; 12%), and warning labels (n = 3; 5%). Local policies in

5 focus areas had a 100% probability of enactment: healthy checkout (n = 2), healthy procurement (n = 9), healthy retail (n = 2), nutrition standards (n = 21), and restaurant children's meals (n = 26). The probability of enactment for warning labels was 75% (of 4), 70% for excise taxes (of 10), and 50% for sales taxes (of 2). Of 26 local-level enacted restaurant children's meals policies, 24 were healthy default beverage policies (Appendix B). Three enacted local-level policies were subsequently repealed: the 2015 Davis, California, restaurant children's meal policy (now under California Senate Bill 1192 [Appendix B]); 2016 San Francisco, California, warning label policy; and 2017 Cook County, Illinois, sales tax policy.

The Tribal policies were the 2014 Navajo Nation sales tax policy and the 2016 Lower Sioux Indian Community nutrition standards policy, both enacted (Appendix B).

Trends in Proposed Policies Over Time

Trends in unique proposed policies by year (2014–2022) and focus area are illustrated in Figures 2 and 3 (2023 was excluded because of the search cutoff date being May 31, 2023, and thus not capturing the full year). Across jurisdictions, the highest number of policies (n = 72) were proposed in 2017, consisting largely of tax (n = 21 excise and n = 3 sales) and restaurant children's meal (n = 11) policies. The highest number of policies were enacted in 2016 (n = 17), consisting mostly of nutrition standards (n = 7) and tax (n = 4 excise; n = 1 sales) policies. The lowest number of policies were proposed in 2022 (n = 12), and lowest number enacted in 2019 and 2022 (n = 5 each). In 2020, the first year of the COVID-19 pandemic, the number of proposed policies (n = 26) decreased by 48% from 2019 (n = 50).

At the state level, the highest number of policies (n = 60) were proposed in 2017, with the largest proportion being tax policies (n = 18 excise; n = 3 sales). The highest number of state-level policies were enacted in 2015 (n = 6: 2 education and outreach, 1 nutrition standards, 1 healthy procurement, 1 research and evaluation, 1 restaurant children's meals; Appendix A, Figure B).

The number of proposed and enacted local excise tax policies decreased after the enactment of state-level preemption laws prohibiting local SSB taxes in 2017 in Michigan, and 2018 in Arizona, California, and Washington.[21,22] Just 1 local excise tax policy (0 enacted) was proposed in 2019 to 2022 compared with 8 (7 enacted) in 2014 to 2018 (Appendix A, Figure C). However, state-level excise tax policies continued to be proposed (n = 52; 0 enacted) in 2017 to 2022 (Appendix A, Figure B).

Density of Proposed Policies by Jurisdiction

California had the highest density of unique policies with 51 proposed policies (state level: n = 24 with 9 [38%] enacted; local level: n = 27 with 26 [96%] enacted; Figure 4). New York State had the next highest policy density with 43 proposed policies (state level: n = 35 with 0 enacted; local level: n = 8 with 8 [100%] enacted). In California, most proposed policies were in 4 focus areas: excise tax (n = 11; 21%), restaurant children's meals (n = 10; 20%), nutrition standards (n = 8; 16%), and warning labels (n = 5; 10%). In New York, most proposed policies were warning labels (n = 11; 26%), restaurant children's meals (n = 10; 23%), nutrition standards (n = 7; 16%), and healthy procurement and excise tax (n = 6 each; 14% each; Appendix B).

DISCUSSION

To our knowledge, this is the first comprehensive inventory of US SSB policies, which includes policies proposed and enacted January 2014 to May 2023. There were 335 state-level (n = 256 unique), 63 local-level, and 2 Tribal-level policies. A higher proportion of local-level policies were enacted than state-level policies. Across levels, the most frequently proposed focus areas included excise taxes, restaurant children's meals, nutrition standards, SNAP, and warning label policies. Among enacted policies, the most frequent focus areas were restaurant children's meals, nutrition standards, education and outreach, healthy procurement, and excise taxes. However, excise taxes, healthy checkout, healthy retail, and warning label policies were enacted only at the local level, despite excise taxes being the most frequently proposed state-level policy. Education and outreach policies made up the largest share (43%) of enacted state-level policies but 0% of proposed and enacted local-level policies. More SSB policies were proposed and enacted in California and New York than in any other state, and policies were proposed more often in 2017 and enacted in 2016 than any other year.

Researchers, policymakers, advocates, and practitioners can use this inventory to understand the SSB policy landscape, conduct additional research on SSB policies, and inform public health advocacy efforts. The inventory includes direct Web links to policies, a policy's proposal and enactment

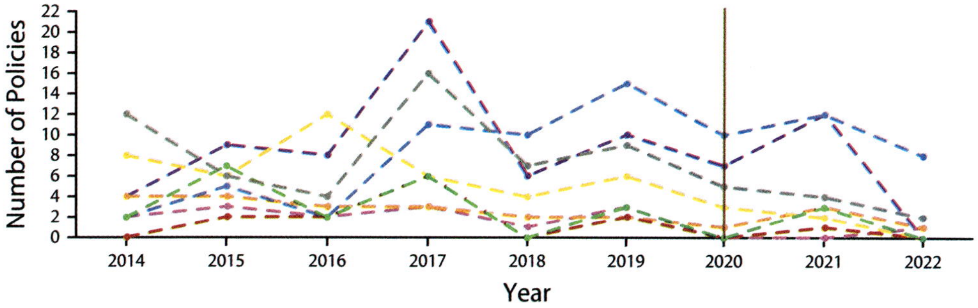

	2014	2015	2016	2017	2018	2019	2020	2021	2022
Excise tax total proposed policies	4	9	8	21	6	10	7	12	0
Sales tax total proposed policies	2	3	2	3	1	3	0	0	1
Healthy procurement total proposed policies	4	4	3	3	2	2	1	3	1
Marketing and advertising total proposed policies	0	2	2	6	0	2	0	1	0
Nutrition standards total proposed policies	8	6	12	6	4	6	3	2	0
Restaurant children's meals total proposed policies	2	5	2	11	10	15	10	12	8
Warning labels total proposed policies	2	7	2	6	0	3	0	3	0
Other total proposed policies	12	6	4	16	7	9	5	4	2
Total policies per year	34	42	35	72	30	50	26	37	12

FIGURE 2— Trends in Total Proposed Sugar-Sweetened Beverage Policies by Year and Focus Area: United States, 2014–2022

Note. Total represents all included unique proposed policies at the local, state, and Tribal levels (i.e., companion policies were counted as a single unique policy, and each focus area of policies with multiple focus areas was counted as a unique policy). Focus areas included in "Other" are education and outreach, healthy checkout, healthy retail, research and evaluation, Supplemental Nutrition Assistance Program (SNAP), size, and water policies. Policies from 2023 are not shown as our policy search concluded in May 2023. Vertical line indicates the year the COVID-19 pandemic began.

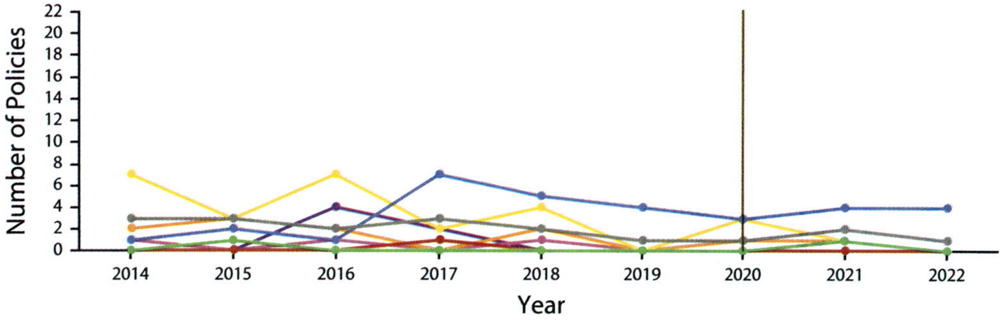

	2014	2015	2016	2017	2018	2019	2020	2021	2022
Excise tax policies enacted	1	0	4	2	0	0	0	0	0
Sales tax policies enacted	1	0	1	0	1	0	0	0	0
Healthy procurement policies enacted	2	3	2	0	2	0	1	1	0
Marketing and advertising policies enacted	0	0	0	1	0	0	0	0	0
Nutrition standards policies enacted	7	3	7	2	4	0	3	1	0
Restaurant children's meals enacted	1	2	1	7	5	4	3	4	4
Warning labels policies enacted	0	1	0	0	0	0	0	1	0
Other policies enacted	3	3	2	3	2	1	1	2	1
Total policies enacted	15	12	17	15	14	5	8	9	5

FIGURE 3— Trends in Total Enacted Sugar-Sweetened Beverage Policies by Year and Focus Area: United States, 2014–2022

Note. Total represents all included unique enacted policies at the local, state, and Tribal levels (i.e., companion policies were counted as a single unique policy and each focus area of policies with multiple focus areas were counted as a unique policy). Focus areas included in "Other" are education and outreach, healthy checkout, healthy retail, research and evaluation, Supplemental Nutrition Assistance Program (SNAP), size, and water policies. Policies from 2023 are not shown as our policy search concluded in May 2023. Vertical line indicates the year the COVID-19 pandemic began.

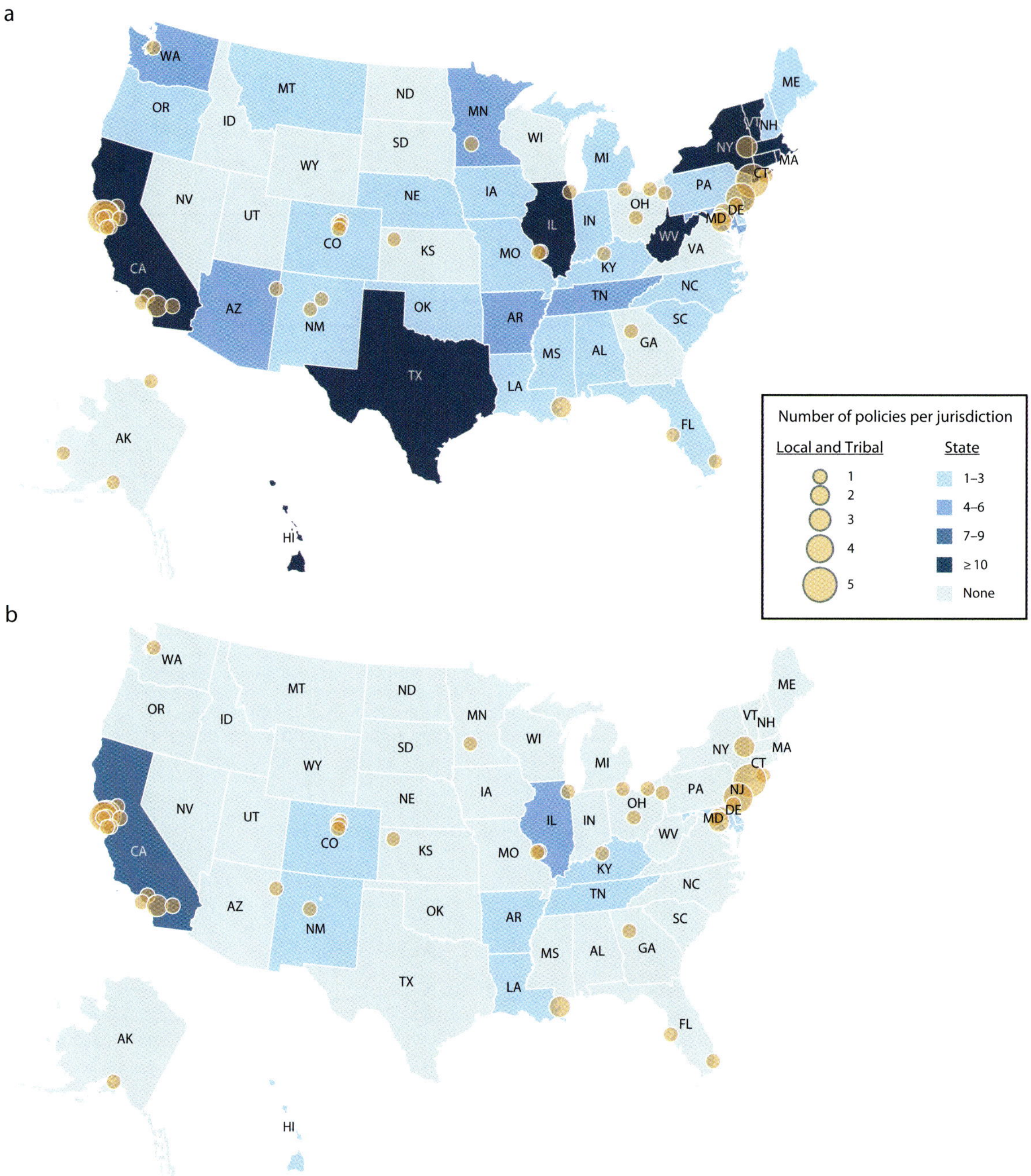

FIGURE 4— **Density of All (a) Proposed and (b) Enacted Policies at State, Local, and Tribal Levels: United States, 2014–2023**

history, and characteristics (e.g., year, status), thus serving as a starting point for policy development and diffusion.

Our study builds upon previous research, including an inventory of US cardiometabolic health policies (2010–2017),[13] a narrative review of select SSB policies,[15] and other studies summarizing SSB legislation in specific areas (e.g., procurement,[23] excise taxes,[11] warning labels,[16] and obesity prevention[24]). Together, our inventory and the extant literature illustrate the potential of SSB policies to reach broad populations while illustrating barriers to adoption.

Trends observed, such as the decrease in policy proposal and enactment since 2019 (except proposal of local-level restaurant children's meals), decrease in local SSB tax proposals, and high rate of enactment of restaurant children's meal policies, should not be interpreted as an indication of policy effectiveness. In fact, some policies that were less likely to be proposed and enacted (e.g., excise taxes [in certain years], warning labels) are among the most (cost) effective.[9,10,25] These trends may reflect barriers like the chilling effect of industry-backed state laws that preempt local SSB taxes, industry-backed SSB tax repeal campaigns (1 of which was successful in Cook County, IL, in 2017), or industry lawsuits and subsequent court decisions (e.g., 9th Circuit Court of Appeals blocking San Francisco's SSB warning label policy). Thus, there may be an overall perceived difficulty (or ease) of policy enactment and perception about the availability of resources for policy advocacy and legal defense.

Trends we observed in the probability of enactment may be inversely related to policy effectiveness because of industry vehemently opposing policies perceived to negatively affect their bottom line.[26] It is particularly notable that only 1 local-level excise tax policy has been proposed since the 2018 preemption laws, given the effectiveness of taxation policies, and that it took, on average, 11 years to repeal tobacco preemption laws.[27] Other influencing factors may include competing priorities (e.g., pandemic), policy novelty, and the interest of funders, the public, community leaders, and policymakers. With the emergency phase of the pandemic concluded and the California preemption landscape evolving, renewed interest in SSB policies could occur. For example, the recent California court ruling that imposing penalties on localities that enact SSB taxes is unconstitutional[28] may lead to revitalized activity in SSB taxes.

As with tobacco-control policies, we observed that the local level served as a laboratory for testing policies, laying the groundwork for dissemination to state and federal levels.[29] For instance, novel and more effective SSB policies (e.g., excise taxes, warning labels, healthy checkout) were enacted only at the local level, while education and outreach policies were enacted only at the state level. Contributing factors may include that education policies have higher acceptance across the political spectrum and lower industry opposition, that states are more politically heterogeneous than cities, or that industry may have less influence over local legislators where accountability to and direct access from local constituents is higher.

Limitations and Strengths

An important limitation of the policy databases used to develop this inventory is the lack of information on Tribal policies. We identified only 2 Tribal policies that fit our inclusion criteria. One was the 2014 Healthy Diné Nation Act, renewed in 2020. In addition to taxing sales of minimal-to-no-nutritional-value foods and beverages, this policy waived a 5% sales tax on healthy foods, with revenue allocated to community wellness projects; as of 2019, 99% of the revenue had been disbursed to Diné Nation health projects.[17] Since implementation, the availability and purchase of healthy food and beverages in the Diné Nation increased.[30] The second was the Lower Sioux Indian Community's Honoring Little Crow with Healthy and Indigenous Foods Initiative (2016), which aimed to improve healthy food and beverage access at community vending machines and events. Other policies that did not meet inclusion criteria were the Osage Nation policy (2020) that established procurement standards for Osage Nation–owned or operated property (excluded because the text did not address SSBs) and the Minneapolis American Indian Center healthy beverage policy that prohibited SSBs at Center-sponsored meetings and events (excluded as an institutional policy).

This inventory focused on US policies, but policy innovations globally can inform domestic policy, including front-of-package nutrient labels, which Chile combined with advertising restrictions, resulting in decreased SSB purchases.[9] In 2020, 2 Mexican states banned sales of SSBs and junk food to minors, and in 2022,[31] the United Kingdom implemented a policy restricting promotion and placement of SSBs and other foods high in saturated fat, sugar, and salt in prominent store locations like end-of-aisle and checkouts.[32] In addition, there are novel SSB policies that have yet to be introduced, like minimum-pricing or proportional-pricing mandates for SSBs, strengthening standards for SNAP-authorized retailers around promotion and placement, implementing a standardized definition of a child-sized SSBs in restaurants, or restricting marketing of harmful foods and beverages in public spaces, government property (including public universities), and online platforms.[14,33,34]

This study's primary strength is that it created the only existing comprehensive database, to our knowledge, of US SSB policies over the last decade and across multiple jurisdictions. The included supplemental table (Appendix B) of policy characteristics and direct Web links can be used by multiple stakeholders to further study, develop, and diffuse policies.

Limitations include the exclusion of federal policies, found elsewhere.[8,13]

We also excluded potentially relevant policies with vague language regarding SSBs (e.g., "healthy beverage" without defining "healthy"), which could make our policy count conservative. We did not include draft policies not (yet) formally proposed, (e.g., a local-level healthy checkout policy from Contra Costa County, CA). In addition, we are likely missing relevant local and Tribal policies, for which there is no comprehensive database, although our survey of experts helped identify missed policies. Lastly, the policy search was not updated past May 2023. Future research is needed to characterize the finer details of policies (e.g., tax rate, type of warning), including studying predictors of policy effectiveness and likelihood of enactment.

Public Health Implications

This study provides the first comprehensive inventory of US SSB policies at the state, local, and Tribal levels from 2014 to 2023, which may be useful for public health officials, policymakers, legal epidemiologists, practitioners, and advocates who are developing SSB policies and who wish to understand the current policy landscape. AJPH

ABOUT THE AUTHORS

Jennie N. Davis is with the Institute for Global Nutrition, University of California, Davis. Shatabdi Goon, Sarah E. Solar, and Jennifer Falbe are with the Department of Human Ecology, University of California, Davis. Jessie Gouck is with the Nutrition and Physical Activity Branch in the Center for Healthy Communities with the California Department of Public Health, Sacramento. Sally Mancini is with the UConn Rudd Center for Food Policy and Health, Hartford, CT. Alberto M. Ortega Hinojosa is an independent researcher, Berkeley, CA. James Krieger is with the School of Public Health, University of Washington, Seattle, WA.

CORRESPONDENCE

Correspondence should be sent to Jennie N. Davis, 3253 Meyer Hall, One Shields Ave, Davis, CA, 95616-5270 (e-mail: jnidavis@ucdavis.edu).

Reprints can be ordered at https://www.ajph.org by clicking the "Reprints" link.

PUBLICATION INFORMATION

Full Citation: Davis JN, Goon S, Gouck J, et al. An inventory of proposed and enacted sugar-sweetened beverage policies at the state, local, and Tribal levels in the United States, 2014–2023. *Am J Public Health*. 2024;114(12):1344–1353.

Acceptance Date: August 16, 2024.

DOI: https://doi.org/10.2105/AJPH.2024.307855

ORCID iDs:

Jennie N. Davis https://orcid.org/0000-0002-2000-8873

Sarah E. Solar https://orcid.org/0000-0003-3423-5708

James Krieger https://orcid.org/0000-0003-4462-9428

Jennifer Falbe https://orcid.org/0000-0002-8405-4326

CONTRIBUTORS

J. N. Davis, J. Gouck, and J. Falbe designed the research. J. N. Davis, S. Goon, S. E. Solar, and J. Falbe conducted the research. J. N. Davis, S. Goon, S. E, Solar, A. M. Ortega Hinojosa, and J. Falbe analyzed the data. S. Goon, S. E. Solar, J. Gouck, S. Mancini, J. Krieger, and J. Falbe provided critical feedback. J. N. Davis wrote the article. J. Falbe had primary responsibility for final content. All authors read and approved the final article.

ACKNOWLEDGMENTS

This study was conducted as part of a contract with the California Department of Public Health with funding from US Department of Agriculture's (USDA's) Supplemental Nutrition Assistance Program Education. J. Falbe was additionally supported by USDA/National Institute of Food and Agriculture (NIFA) Hatch project 7005204, and the National Institute of Diabetes and Digestive and Kidney Diseases of the National Institutes of Health under award K01DK113068.

We would like to thank the following people and entities for providing additional local policies and insights: Sarah H. Mann and the American Heart Association, Center for Science in the Public Interest, and Sabrina Adler and ChangeLab Solutions. We would also like to thank Angelique EagleWoman, JD, LLM, of the Native American Law and Sovereignty Institute, Mitchell Hamline School of Law, for her guidance and insight on Tribal policy nomenclature. Finally, we would like to acknowledge the research support of the following staff and students: Kris Jayme Matas, Kathy Pham, GeAnn Santos, and Ethan Christopher Wolf.

Note. The findings, content, and conclusions in this article are those of the author(s) and do not necessarily represent the views or opinions of the California Department of Public Health, the California Health and Human Services Agency, the USDA/NIFA, or the National Institutes of Health.

CONFLICTS OF INTEREST

All authors report no conflicts of interest.

HUMAN PARTICIPANT PROTECTION

This study involved non–human participant research, and institutional review board approval was not required.

REFERENCES

1. Lloyd-Jones DM, Hong Y, Labarthe D, et al. Defining and setting national goals for cardiovascular health promotion and disease reduction. *Circulation*. 2010;121(4):586–613. https://doi.org/10.1161/CIRCULATIONAHA.109.192703
2. *Guideline: Sugars Intake for Adults and Children*. Geneva, Switzerland: World Health Organization; 2015.
3. Drewnowski A, Rehm CD. Consumption of added sugars among US children and adults by food purchase location and food source. *Am J Clin Nutr*. 2014;100(3):901–907. https://doi.org/10.3945/ajcn.114.089458
4. Malik VS, Hu FB. The role of sugar-sweetened beverages in the global epidemics of obesity and chronic diseases. *Nat Rev Endocrinol*. 2022;18(4):205–218. https://doi.org/10.1038/s41574-021-00627-6
5. Bleich SN, Vercammen KA. The negative impact of sugar-sweetened beverages on children's health: an update of the literature. *BMC Obes*. 2018;5(1):6. https://doi.org/10.1186/s40608-017-0178-9
6. Kaplan S, White JS, Madsen KA, Basu S, Villas-Boas SB, Schillinger D. Evaluation of changes in prices and purchases following implementation of sugar-sweetened beverage taxes across the US. *JAMA Health Forum*. 2024;5(1):e234737. https://doi.org/10.1001/jamahealthforum.2023.4737
7. Andreyeva T, Marple K, Marinello S, Moore TE, Powell LM. Outcomes following taxation of sugar-sweetened beverages: a systematic review and meta-analysis. *JAMA Netw Open*. 2022;5(6):e2215276. https://doi.org/10.1001/jamanetworkopen.2022.15276
8. Krieger J, Bleich SN, Scarmo S, Ng SW. Sugar-sweetened beverage reduction policies: progress and promise. *Annu Rev Public Health*. 2021;42(1):439–461. https://doi.org/10.1146/annurev-publhealth-090419-103005
9. Taillie LS, Reyes M, Colchero MA, Popkin B, Corvalán C. An evaluation of Chile's Law of Food Labeling and Advertising on sugar-sweetened beverage purchases from 2015 to 2017: a before-and-after study. *PLoS Med*. 2020;17(2):e1003015. https://doi.org/10.1371/journal.pmed.1003015
10. Wilde P, Huang Y, Sy S, et al. Cost-effectiveness of a US national sugar-sweetened beverage tax with a multistakeholder approach: who pays and who benefits. *Am J Public Health*. 2019;109(2):276–284. https://doi.org/10.2105/AJPH.2018.304803
11. Krieger J, Magee K, Hennings T, Schoof J, Madsen KA. How sugar-sweetened beverage tax revenues are being used in the United States. *Prev Med Rep*. 2021;23:101388. https://doi.org/10.1016/j.pmedr.2021.101388

12. Falbe J. The ethics of excise taxes on sugar-sweetened beverages. *Physiol Behav.* 2020; 225:113105. https://doi.org/10.1016/j.physbeh.2020.113105
13. Huang Y, Pomeranz J, Wilde P, et al. Adoption and design of emerging dietary policies to improve cardiometabolic health in the US. *Curr Atheroscler Rep.* 2018;20(5):25. https://doi.org/10.1007/s11883-018-0726-x
14. Pomeranz JL, Miller DP. Policies to promote healthy portion sizes for children. *Appetite.* 2015;88:50–58. https://doi.org/10.1016/j.appet.2014.12.003
15. Falbe J, Madsen K. Growing momentum for sugar-sweetened beverage campaigns and policies: costs and considerations. *Am J Public Health.* 2017;107(6):835–838. https://doi.org/10.2105/AJPH.2017.303805
16. Pomeranz JL, Mozaffarian D, Micha R. Sugar-sweetened beverage warning policies in the broader legal context: health and safety warning laws and the First Amendment. *Am J Prev Med.* 2020;58(6):783–788. https://doi.org/10.1016/j.amepre.2020.01.006
17. Yazzie D, Tallis K, Curley C, et al. The Navajo Nation Healthy Diné Nation Act: a description of community wellness projects funded by a 2% tax on minimal-to-no-nutritious-value foods. *J Public Health Manag Pract.* 2022;28(2):E471–E479. https://doi.org/10.1097/PHH.0000000000001371
18. Au LE, Ritchie LD, Gurzo K, et al. Post-Healthy, Hunger-Free Kids Act adherence to select school nutrition standards by region and poverty level: the Healthy Communities Study. *J Nutr Educ Behav.* 2020;52(3):249–258. https://doi.org/10.1016/j.jneb.2019.10.016
19. Hopkins LC, Gunther C. A historical review of changes in nutrition standards of USDA child meal programs relative to research findings on the nutritional adequacy of program meals and the diet and nutritional health of participants: implications for future research and the summer food service program. *Nutrients.* 2015;7(12): 10145–10167. https://doi.org/10.3390/nu7125523
20. Schwartz MB, Brownell KD, Miller DL. Primer on US food and nutrition policy and public health: protect school nutrition standards. *Am J Public Health.* 2019;109(7):990–991. https://doi.org/10.2105/AJPH.2019.305072
21. Falbe J, Adler SS, Roberto CA. Sugar-sweetened beverage tax preemption and the urgency of unified mobilization. *Am J Public Health.* 2021;111(4): 546–548. https://doi.org/10.2105/AJPH.2021.306163
22. Crosbie E, Pomeranz JL, Wright KE, Hoeper S, Schmidt L. State preemption: an emerging threat to local sugar-sweetened beverage taxation. *Am J Public Health.* 2021;111(4):677–686. https://doi.org/10.2105/AJPH.2020.306062
23. Lowry-Warnock A, Strombom N, Mugavero K, Harris D, Blanck HM, Onufrak S. Advancing healthy food service in the United States: state food service guidelines policy adoption and implementation supports, 2015–2019. *Am J Health Promot.* 2023;37(3):300–312. https://doi.org/10.1177/08901171221123311
24. Donaldson EA, Cohen JE, Villanti AC, Kanarek NF, Barry CL, Rutkow L. Patterns and predictors of state adult obesity prevention legislation enactment in US states: 2010–2013. *Prev Med.* 2015; 74:117–122. https://doi.org/10.1016/j.ypmed.2015.02.013
25. Lee Y, Mozaffarian D, Sy S, et al. Health impact and cost-effectiveness of volume, tiered, and absolute sugar content sugar-sweetened beverage tax policies in the United States. *Circulation.* 2020;142(6):523–534. https://doi.org/10.1161/CIRCULATIONAHA.119.042956
26. Pfister K. Leaked: Coca-Cola's worldwide political strategy to kill soda taxes. *Medium.* October 27, 2017. Available at: https://medium.com/cokeleak/leaked-coca-colas-worldwide-political-strategy-to-kill-soda-taxes-9717f361fb04. Accessed March 13, 2024.
27. Crosbie E, Schmidt LA. Preemption in tobacco control: a framework for other areas of public health. *Am J Public Health.* 2020;110(3):345–350. https://doi.org/10.2105/AJPH.2019.305473
28. *Cultiva La Salud v State of California*. Justia Law. March 22, 2024. Available at: https://law.justia.com/cases/california/court-of-appeal/2023/c095486.html. Accessed March 13, 2024.
29. Francis JA, Abramsohn EM, Park HY. Policy-driven tobacco control. *Tob Control.* 2010;19(suppl 1):i16–i20. https://doi.org/10.1136/tc.2009.030718
30. George C, Bancroft C, Salt SK, et al. Changes in food pricing and availability on the Navajo Nation following a 2% tax on unhealthy foods: The Healthy Diné Nation Act of 2014. *PLoS One.* 2021;16(9):e0256683. https://doi.org/10.1371/journal.pone.0256683
31. Fredrick J. Mexican states ban sale of junk food to minors. NPR. September 5, 2020. Available at: https://www.npr.org/2020/09/05/909969074/mexico-bans-sale-of-junk-food-to-minors. Accessed December 8, 2023.
32. Muir S, Dhuria P, Roe E, Lawrence W, Baird J, Vogel C. UK government's new placement legislation is a 'good first step': a rapid qualitative analysis of consumer, business, enforcement and health stakeholder perspectives. *BMC Med.* 2023;21(1):33. https://doi.org/10.1186/s12916-023-02726-9
33. Harris JL, Webb V, Sacco SJ, Pomeranz JL. Marketing to children in supermarkets: an opportunity for public policy to improve children's diets. *Int J Environ Res Public Health.* 2020;17(4):1284. https://doi.org/10.3390/ijerph17041284
34. Pamukcu A, Peters M. *Sugary Drink Strategy Playbook: Reducing Sugary Drinks to Promote Community Health and Equity*. ChangeLab Solutions. 2018. Available at: https://www.changelabsolutions.org/product/sugary-drink-strategy-playbook. Accessed May 24, 2023.

Countermarketing Versus Health Education Messages About Sugar-Sweetened Beverages: An Online Randomized Controlled Trial of US Adults

Anna H. Grummon, PhD, MSPH, Amanda B. Zeitlin, MPH, Cristina J. Y. Lee, MPH, Marissa G. Hall, PhD, MSPH, Caroline Collis, BA, Lauren P. Cleveland, MS, MPH, and Joshua Petimar, ScD

See also State Laws Targeting Marginalized Groups, pp. 1322–1353.

Objectives. To test whether countermarketing messages for sugary drinks lead to lower intentions to consume sugary drinks and less perceived weight stigma than health education messages.

Methods. In August 2023, we conducted an online randomized controlled trial with US adults (n = 2169). We assessed the effect of countermarketing messages, health education messages, and neutral control messages on intentions to consume sugary drinks and perceived weight stigma.

Results. Both countermarketing messages (Cohen $d = -0.20$) and health education messages ($d = -0.35$) led to lower intentions to consume sugary drinks than control messages ($Ps < .001$). However, both types of messages elicited more perceived weight stigma than control messages ($ds = 0.87$ and 1.29, respectively; $Ps < .001$). Countermarketing messages were less effective than health education messages at lowering intentions to consume sugary drinks (d for countermarketing vs health education = 0.14) but also elicited less perceived weight stigma than health education messages ($d = -0.39$; $Ps < .01$).

Conclusions. Countermarketing messages show promise for reducing sugary drink consumption while eliciting less weight stigma than health education messages, though they may need to be refined further to minimize weight stigma and maximize effectiveness.

Clinical Trial Number. ClinicalTrials.gov NCT05953194. (*Am J Public Health*. 2024;114(12):1354–1364. https://doi.org/10.2105/AJPH.2024.307853)

AJPH December 2024, Vol. 114, No. 12

Consuming sugary drinks increases risk of heart disease, high blood pressure, type 2 diabetes, and tooth decay.[1] Despite some declines in sugary drink consumption over the last decade, nearly two thirds of adults in the United States consume at least 1 sugary drink every day,[1] suggesting that new strategies are needed to reduce sugary drink consumption. Media campaigns (including those delivered through print, broadcast, and social media) are a highly scalable strategy for increasing knowledge, shifting attitudes and norms, and ultimately encouraging people to adopt healthier behaviors,[2] including limiting sugary drink consumption.[3–5]

Most sugary drink media campaigns are health education campaigns that contain messages seeking to reduce sugary drink consumption by educating consumers about the health harms of sugary drinks.[3] Recently, however, researchers and health departments have begun to develop a new approach to sugary drink media campaigns borrowed from tobacco control: countermarketing.[3,6] Countermarketing campaigns seek to reduce consumption of unhealthy products by exposing and undermining deceptive, manipulative, misleading, or harmful marketing activities used by the companies that make them.[6] Countermarketing campaigns have been successfully used to reduce smoking,[6] prompting researchers to begin applying countermarketing to discourage people from consuming unhealthy foods and beverages.[7–10] Although few real-world countermarketing campaigns for sugary drinks have been evaluated, 2 studies found that parents exposed to these campaigns had lower intentions to serve sugary drinks and were less likely to select sugary drinks for their children compared with parents exposed to control campaigns not about beverages.[11,12]

As interest grows in using countermarketing campaigns to reduce sugary drink consumption, it is important to compare messages for countermarketing campaigns to messages for health education campaigns on both effectiveness and unintended consequences. One potential advantage of countermarketing messages is that they are designed to counteract the effects of sugary drink marketing,[6] whereas health education messages typically do not address marketing. Sugary drink marketing uses positive, emotional messaging to encourage consumers to develop lasting positive attitudes toward marketed brands[7] and purchase more sugary drinks.[8] Countermarketing messages aim to undermine the effects of marketing by exposing marketing practices that are deceptive, manipulative, misleading, or harmful. For example, the Hawaii Department of Health's "Sweet Lies" countermarketing campaign exposes how companies put marketing claims like "natural" and "100% vitamin C" on fruit-flavored drinks to mislead consumers into thinking these drinks are healthier than they are.[9] By exposing deceptive, manipulative, misleading, and harmful marketing practices, countermarketing messages increase negative attitudes toward sugary drink companies and, in turn, reduce sugary drink consumption. Moreover, by exposing these marketing practices, countermarketing messages may be especially motivating to young adults, who tend to be more motivated by proximal outcomes (like not wanting to be manipulated by sugary drink marketing practices) than distal outcomes (like diabetes or heart disease).[10,13]

A second potential advantage of countermarketing messages is that they emphasize industry accountability for body weight, whereas some health education campaigns (implicitly or explicitly) emphasize individual responsibility for body weight. Emphasizing individual responsibility for body weight can lead people to devalue or reject people with higher body weight (i.e., can increase weight stigma).[14] By focusing on industry accountability rather than individual responsibility for body weight, countermarketing messages could elicit less weight stigma than health education campaigns. Minimizing weight stigma is a critical goal for public health campaigns given that weight stigma reduces diet quality and worsens mental and physical health.[15,16]

Despite the potential benefits of countermarketing over health education, few studies have compared adults' responses to countermarketing and health education messages.[3] To address this gap, we examined whether countermarketing messages for sugary drinks lead to lower intentions to consume sugary drinks and less perceived weight stigma than health education messages. We also examined whether countermarketing messages' beneficial effects on intentions are larger among young adults compared with older adults.

METHODS

On August 7, 2023, we recruited a national convenience sample of US adults through the survey company CloudResearch Connect. CloudResearch recruits adults to its panel using online advertisements and word of mouth. CloudResearch uses e-mail and web dashboard invitations to invite panelists to participate in specific research studies.

Participants were eligible for this study if they lived in the United States and were aged 18 years or older. To maximize statistical power to detect moderation by age group, we used quotas to ensure that approximately half of participants were young adults (aged 18–29 years) and half were older adults (aged ≥ 30 years).

Approach

The study was guided by a conceptual model of how countermarketing and health education messages affect behavior (Appendix Figure A, available as a supplement to the online version of this article at https://ajph.org). The study adopted a 3-arm, between-subjects, randomized controlled design. We randomized participants to 1 of 3 trial arms with a 1:1:1 simple allocation ratio: (1) countermarketing messages discouraging sugary drink consumption, (2) health education messages discouraging sugary drink consumption, or (3) control messages (neutral messages about safe driving). The survey software automatically randomized participants. Figure 1 depicts the CONSORT diagram.

Message and Image Design

We developed the text and images for the study based on existing media campaigns and best practices. The countermarketing messages followed principles of effective countermarketing campaigns, including describing industry manipulation of consumers, appealing to emotions, describing health consequences, and criticizing the industry for using targeted marketing.[6] The health education messages focused on describing the sugar content in sugary drinks and the health consequences of sugary drink consumption (e.g., weight gain, diabetes), using text and images adapted from previous campaigns.[3] The control messages were matched to the countermarketing and health education messages on length, but discussed a neutral topic unrelated to sugary drinks (safe driving), similar to a previous study.[11] The control messages were adapted from messages created by the National Highway Traffic Safety Administration. All messages were presented as Instagram posts to increase realism. Messages were matched for approximate length across the 3 trial arms (27–49 words each, including words in the main image plus the caption). We did not conduct formal pretesting of the messages. Sample messages and images are shown in Figure 2, and all messages and images are shown in Appendix Figure B.

Procedures

Participants provided electronic informed consent and completed an online survey programmed in Qualtrics. Participants first answered unrelated survey questions about environmental sustainability labels for a separate study, then completed the randomized trial for the present study. For the present study, participants viewed the 3 messages from their randomly assigned arm 1 at a time (displayed in order, see Appendix Figure B). The survey displayed each message for

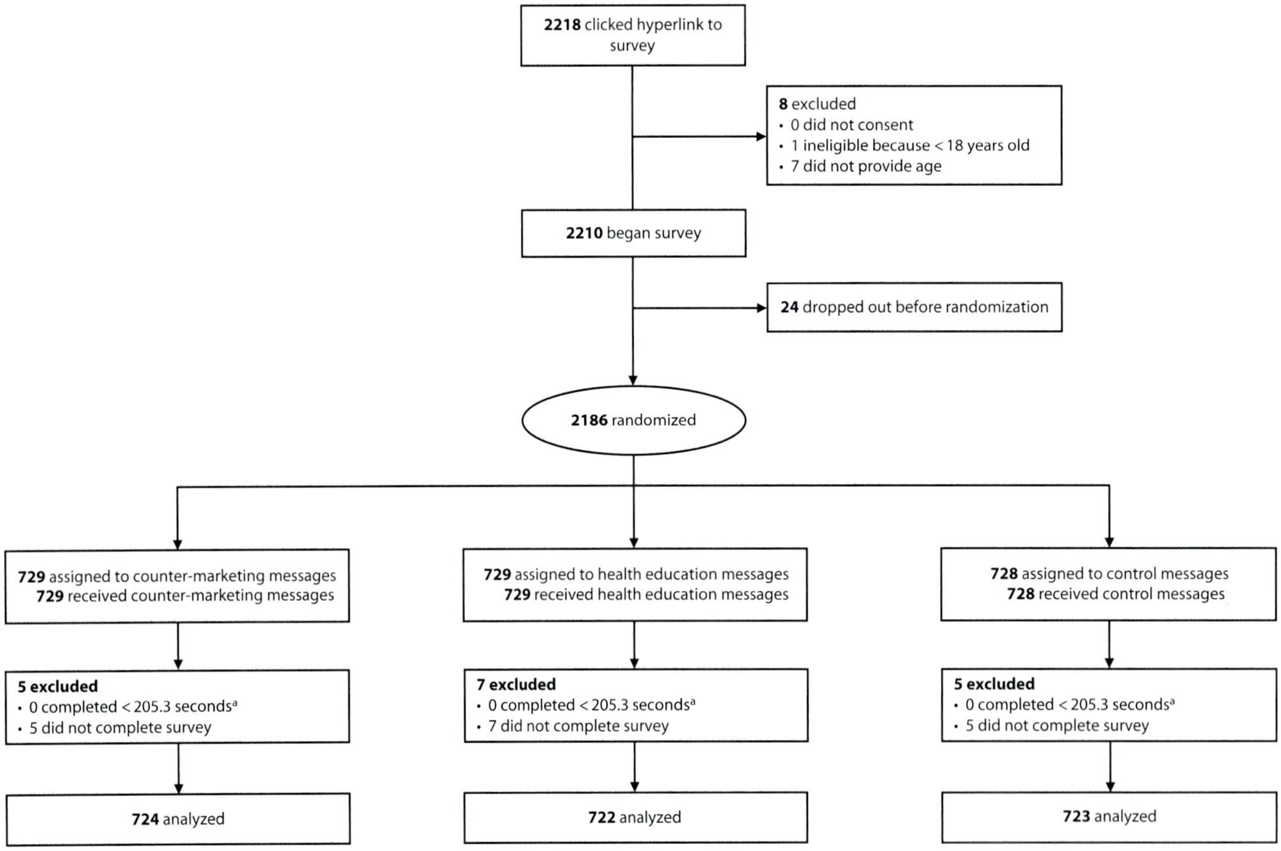

FIGURE 1— CONSORT Flow Diagram

[a]One third of median completion time (median = 10 minutes, 16 seconds).

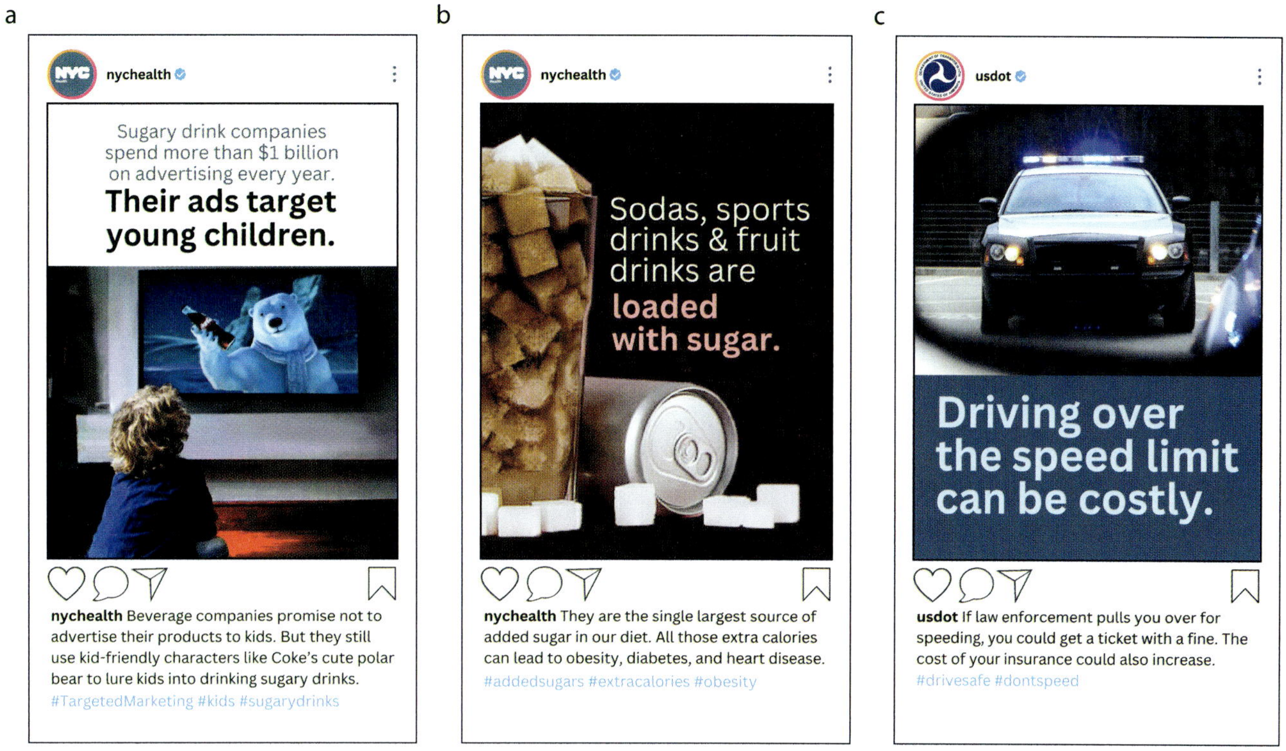

FIGURE 2— Example Messages and Images Used in the Trial for (a) Countermarketing Messages Discouraging Sugary Drink Consumption, (b) Health Education Messages Discouraging Sugary Drink Consumption, and (c) Control Messages (Neutral Messages About Safe Driving)

Note. All messages and images are shown in Appendix Figure B (available as a supplement to the online version of this article at https://ajph.org).

10 seconds before participants could advance to the next message. After viewing their messages, participants answered survey questions as described in the next section.

Measures

The primary outcome was intentions to consume sugary drinks. We focused on intentions because a meta-analysis of experiments demonstrated that changing intentions leads to changes in behavior.[17] We assessed intentions to consume sugary drinks with 2 items[18] (e.g., "In the next week, I plan to drink sugary drinks like sodas, sports drinks, or fruit drinks").

Guided by our conceptual model, the survey also assessed 4 sets of secondary outcomes. First, we assessed perceived weight stigma of the messages using 3 items[19] (e.g., "These messages increase blame towards people for being overweight"). Second, we assessed 3 message reactions: perceived message effectiveness for discouraging sugary drink consumption, negative feelings about consuming sugary drinks, and anticipated social interactions, each assessed with 1 item.[18,20] Third, we assessed negative attitudes toward sugary drink companies using 1 item.[21] Fourth, we assessed message reactance (i.e., opposition to messages because of feelings that one's autonomy is being threatened) using 2 items.[22] We excluded anger toward the message from our measure of message reactance because including it substantially reduced internal consistency: Cronbach α including anger = 0.49; Spearman–Brown reliability coefficient excluding anger = 0.69. Response options for all items ranged from low (coded as 1) to high (coded as 5). We selected these outcomes because they may be indicative of messages' potential to elicit long-term behavior change.[17,23,24] We show all survey items in Appendix Table A.

Finally, the survey assessed participant characteristics including potential moderators such as age, gender, trait reactance (i.e., a predisposition to perceiving situations as threatening one's freedom[25]), body mass index (BMI, defined as weight in kilograms divided by the square of height in meters [kg/m^2]), and perceived weight status.[26]

Analysis

We preregistered the analysis plan before data collection (https://aspredicted.org/HY8_KVV). We used ordinary least squares regression, regressing each outcome on indicator variables for trial arm (excluding the control as the referent). We used the models to estimate average differential effects (i.e., differences in predicted means between arms) for the countermarketing and health education arms versus the control arm and to test whether the effects of the countermarketing and health education arms differed from one another. We also converted the average differential effects to Cohen *d*s (i.e., standardized effects) to interpret whether differences were small ($d = 0.20$), medium ($d = 0.50$), or large ($d = 0.80$).[27]

We conducted 3 sets of planned exploratory moderation analyses (all preregistered except where noted). First, we examined whether the effects of trial arm on intentions to consume sugary drinks were moderated by age, gender, race, ethnicity, educational attainment, income, or trait reactance (the race, ethnicity, education, and income tests were not preregistered). Second, we examined whether the effects of trial arm on perceived weight stigma were moderated by gender, BMI, or perceived weight status. Third, we examined whether the effects of trial arm on message reactance were moderated by age, gender, or trait reactance. Moderation analyses used the same model as the main analyses with additional terms for the moderator and interactions between the moderator and the trial arms. For all moderation analyses, we tested for moderation by examining the joint significance of the coefficients on all interaction terms and report the effect of the countermarketing and health education messages at each level of the categorical moderators and at the mean plus or minus 1 standard deviation of the continuous moderators.

Previous studies of countermarketing messages have found effects on sugary drink intentions or selection of approximately Cohen $d = 0.2$ to 0.4.[11,13] To be conservative, we estimated sample size needs to detect a somewhat smaller standardized effect size of $d = 0.15$. Analyses indicated that a sample size of 2097 participants (699 per arm) would provide 80% power to detect a standardized difference between arms of Cohen $d = 0.15$ or larger, assuming $\alpha = 0.05$. To account for potential missing data, we aimed to recruit approximately 2150 participants. Per the preregistration, analyses excluded participants who did not complete the survey, yielding an analytic sample of 2169 participants (Figure 1).

All analyses used 2-tailed statistical tests with $\alpha = 0.05$. Analyses were conducted in Stata version 18 (StataCorp LLC, College Station, TX) and were replicated by a second analyst.

RESULTS

Approximately half (49%) of participants were young adults (aged 18–29 years), consistent with recruitment goals (Table 1). Approximately 71% identified as White, 12% as Black or African American, 9% as Asian or Pacific Islander, 6% as other or multiracial, and 1% as American Indian or Alaskan Native. Approximately one third (34%) had educational attainment of some college or less, and 36% had a household income less than $50 000 per year. Compared with the US population, the sample had a higher proportion of young adults (consistent with recruitment goals), people identifying as White or Asian or Pacific Islander, people with a college degree, and people with a household income less than $75 000, and a lower proportion of people identifying as Latino and with a household income of $75 000 or more (Appendix Table B).

Intentions to Consume Sugary Drinks

Both the countermarketing messages (difference vs control = −0.27; 95% confidence interval [CI] = −0.40, –0.13; $P < .001$; Cohen $d = -0.20$) and health education messages (difference vs control = −0.45; 95% CI = −0.58, –0.31; $P < .001$; $d = -0.35$) led to lower intentions to consume sugary drinks than the control messages (Table 2). The effect of the countermarketing messages on intentions to consume sugary drinks was weaker than the effect of the health education messages (difference, countermarketing vs health education = 0.18; 95% CI = 0.05, 0.31; $P = .009$; $d = 0.14$).

We did not observe evidence that the effect of trial arm on intentions to consume sugary drinks was moderated by gender, race, ethnicity, educational attainment, income, or trait reactance (all *P*s for interactions > 0.44; Appendix Table C). Similarly, the interaction terms for age did not reach statistical significance (*P* for interaction = 0.08), though the descriptive pattern suggested potential differences by age. Among older adults (≥ 30 years), the countermarketing messages appeared to have a weaker effect on intentions to consume sugary drinks than the health education messages (differences vs control = −0.31; 95% CI = −0.50, –0.12; $d = -0.23$ and −0.60; 95% CI = −0.79, –0.41; $d = -0.45$, respectively; Appendix Table C). By contrast,

AJPH December 2024, Vol. 114, No. 12

TABLE 1— Participant Characteristics in an Online Randomized Controlled Trial of Countermarketing, Health Education, and Control Messages: United States, 2023

Characteristic	Countermarketing Messages (n = 724), No. (%)	Health Education Messages (n = 722), No. (%)	Control Messages (n = 723), No. (%)
Age, y			
18–29	360 (50)	362 (50)	350 (48)
30–44	236 (33)	219 (30)	236 (33)
45–59	89 (12)	93 (13)	98 (14)
≥ 60	39 (5)	48 (7)	39 (5)
Gender			
Woman	341 (47)	339 (47)	323 (45)
Man	361 (50)	369 (51)	388 (54)
Nonbinary or another gender	22 (3)	14 (2)	12 (2)
Race			
American Indian/Alaska Native	7 (1)	14 (2)	8 (1)
Asian or Pacific Islander	70 (10)	64 (9)	70 (10)
Black or African American	100 (14)	89 (12)	77 (11)
White	486 (67)	510 (71)	535 (74)
Other or multiracial	61 (8)	45 (6)	33 (5)
Latino(a) or Hispanic	71 (10)	87 (12)	78 (11)
Education			
High-school diploma or less	104 (14)	89 (12)	96 (13)
Some college	147 (20)	141 (20)	154 (21)
College graduate or associates degree	371 (51)	391 (54)	353 (49)
Graduate degree	102 (14)	101 (14)	120 (17)
Household income, annual, $			
0–24 999	102 (14)	96 (13)	95 (13)
25 000–49 999	154 (21)	179 (25)	163 (23)
50 000–74 999	149 (21)	159 (22)	147 (20)
≥ 75 000	318 (44)	288 (40)	318 (44)
Household size			
1–2	337 (47)	355 (49)	334 (46)
3–4	299 (41)	295 (41)	308 (43)
≥ 5	88 (12)	72 (10)	81 (11)
No. of children			
0	477 (66)	497 (69)	485 (67)
1–2	212 (29)	198 (27)	206 (28)
≥ 3	35 (5)	27 (4)	32 (4)
Political party identification			
Democrat	424 (59)	389 (54)	411 (57)
Republican	170 (23)	180 (25)	168 (23)
Independent or other	130 (18)	153 (21)	144 (20)

Note. The sample size was n = 2169 US adults. Missing data ranged from 0.0% to 0.05%. Percentages may not sum to 100% because of rounding.

TABLE 2— Effects of Health Education Messages and Countermarketing Messages on Intentions, Perceived Weight Stigma, Message Reactions, Negative Attitudes Toward Sugary Drink Companies, and Message Reactance in US Adults, 2023

Outcome	Countermarketing Messages, Mean (SD)	Health Education Messages, Mean (SD)	Control Messages, Mean (SD)	Countermarketing vs Control: ADE (95% CI)	Countermarketing vs Control: *d*	Health Education vs Control: ADE (95% CI)	Health Education vs Control: *d*	Countermarketing vs Health Education: ADE (95% CI)	Countermarketing vs Health Education: *d*
Intentions to consume sugary drinks	2.53 (1.32)	2.35 (1.25)	2.80 (1.33)	−0.27 (−0.40, −0.13)	−0.20	−0.45 (−0.58, −0.31)	−0.35	0.18 (0.05, 0.31)	0.14
Perceived weight stigma	1.93 (1.05)	2.36 (1.13)	1.19 (0.59)	0.74 (0.64, 0.84)	0.87	1.16 (1.07, 1.26)	1.29	−0.43 (−0.53, −0.33)	−0.39
Message reactions									
Perceived message effectiveness for discouraging sugary drinks	3.59 (1.15)	3.94 (1.08)	1.30 (0.79)	2.29 (2.18, 2.39)	2.31	2.63 (2.53, 2.74)	2.79	−0.35 (−0.45, −0.24)	−0.31
Anticipated social interactions about messages	2.42 (1.22)	2.54 (1.25)	1.81 (1.12)	0.61 (0.48, 0.73)	0.52	0.73 (0.61, 0.86)	0.62	−0.13 (−0.25, −0.002)	−0.10
Negative feelings about consuming sugary drinks	4.10 (0.90)	4.33 (0.90)	3.07 (0.54)	1.03 (0.95, 1.11)	1.39	1.26 (1.18, 1.35)	1.71	−0.23 (−0.32, −0.15)	−0.26
Negative attitudes about sugary drink companies	3.44 (0.91)	3.34 (0.89)	3.09 (0.86)	0.35 (0.26, 0.44)	0.40	0.25 (0.16, 0.35)	0.29	0.10 (0.005, 0.19)	0.11
Message reactance	2.54 (1.02)	2.35 (1.04)	1.91 (0.92)	0.63 (0.53, 0.74)	0.65	0.44 (0.33, 0.54)	0.44	0.20 (0.09, 0.30)	0.19

Note. ADE = average differential effect; CI = confidence interval; *d* = Cohen *d*. The sample size was n = 2169 US adults. There were no missing data on any outcome.

among young adults (aged 18–29 years), the countermarketing messages had similar effects on intentions to consume sugary drinks as the health education messages (differences vs control = −0.23; 95% CI = −0.42, −0.04; *d* = −0.18 and −0.30; 95% CI = −0.49, −0.12; *d* = −0.25, respectively).

Perceived Weight Stigma

Both the countermarketing messages and the health education messages led to higher perceived weight stigma than the control messages (differences vs control = 0.74; 95% CI = 0.64, 0.84; *d* = 0.87 and 1.16; 95% CI = 1.07, 1.26; *d* = 1.29, respectively; both *P*s < .001). The countermarketing messages led to lower perceived weight stigma than the health education messages (difference = −0.43; 95% CI = −0.53, −0.33; *P* < .001; *d* = −0.39).

Effects of the countermarketing and health education messages on perceived weight stigma appeared to be moderated by gender (*P* for interaction < .001), BMI (*P* for interaction = .002), and perceived weight status (*P* for interaction = .07; Appendix Table D). Specifically, the detrimental effects of both the countermarketing and health education messages on perceived weight stigma appeared to be stronger for participants who identified as women compared with men, who reported higher compared with lower BMI, and who perceived themselves to be overweight or (for the health education messages only) underweight compared with those who perceived themselves to be "about the right weight."

Message Reactions

Both the countermarketing messages and the health education messages led to stronger message reactions than the control messages, including higher perceived message effectiveness for discouraging sugary drink consumption, more anticipated social interactions about the messages, and more negative feelings about consuming sugary drinks than the control messages (all $Ps < .001$, Table 2). For all 3 message reactions, the countermarketing messages led to weaker message reactions than the health education messages (all $Ps < .05$).

Negative Attitudes Toward Sugary Drink Companies

Both the countermarketing messages and the health education messages led to more negative attitudes toward sugary drink companies than the control messages ($Ps < .001$; Table 2). The countermarketing messages led to more negative attitudes toward sugary drink companies than the health education messages ($P = .04$).

Message Reactance

Both the countermarketing messages and the health education messages led to higher message reactance than the control messages, with a larger effect for the countermarketing messages (all $Ps < .001$). The effects of the health education and countermarketing messages on message reactance did not appear to be moderated by age, gender, or trait reactance ($Ps > .11$; Appendix Table E).

DISCUSSION

In this online randomized trial with a large national sample of US adults, both countermarketing and health education messages led to lower intentions to consume sugary drinks. Both countermarketing and health education messages, however, elicited more perceived weight stigma than control messages. The countermarketing messages were not as effective as the health education messages in reducing intentions to consume sugary drinks in the overall sample, but they elicited substantially less perceived weight stigma. These results suggest that countermarketing messages could serve as a useful and potentially less-stigmatizing alternative to health education messages for reducing sugary beverage consumption, but they will need to be further refined to maximize their effectiveness and minimize their unintended effects on weight stigma.

Both the countermarketing messages and the health education messages reduced participants' intentions to consume sugary drinks. Both types of messages also increased perceived discouragement from consuming sugary drinks, negative feelings about consuming sugary drinks, and anticipating talking with others about the messages. Because these outcomes can be predictive of behavior change,[17,18,20,23] our results add to the growing body of evidence that exposure to sugary drink messages—whether countermarketing or health education messages—could improve diet-related outcomes.[2,3] Exploratory moderation analyses revealed evidence of potentially differential effects on intentions by age. For older adults, the countermarketing messages appeared to have weaker effects on decreasing intentions to consume sugary drinks than the health education messages. For young adults, however, the countermarketing messages performed similarly to the health education messages. Countermarketing messages may therefore be a promising avenue for improving young adults' dietary behavior, an important finding given that young adults consume more sugary drinks than older adults[1] and that their dietary behaviors track into later adulthood.[28] However, given the exploratory nature of our moderation analyses, replication of this finding is warranted.

Both the health education and the countermarketing messages led to higher perceived weight stigma than the control messages, especially for people who identified as women and those with higher BMI. These findings are potentially concerning given that weight stigma is widespread and harmful to mental and physical health.[15,16] Importantly, the countermarketing messages led to less perceived weight stigma than the health education messages, perhaps because the health education messages focused on the health consequences of sugary drinks. This focus may have implied that individuals are primarily responsible for their body weight,[29] an attribution of responsibility that tends to increase weight stigma.[15] By contrast, the countermarketing messages focused on deceptive, misleading, and harmful industry marketing practices and may therefore have implied that industry is at least partially responsible for body weight.[6] Although more refinement is needed, our results suggest that countermarketing messages may be a strategy for improving diet-related behaviors while reducing harmful unintended effects on weight stigma.

The countermarketing messages elicited stronger negative attitudes toward sugary drink companies than both the control messages and the health education messages, perhaps because they emphasized deceptive industry marketing practices. This finding is important because increasing negative attitudes toward companies could be a mechanism through which countermarketing messages reduce consumption of unhealthy foods and beverages,[30] though it will be challenging to fully counter the persuasive effects of the beverage industry's marketing practices. Still, eliciting negative attitudes toward sugary drink companies could have the additional benefit of boosting the public's support for wider policy changes to reduce sugary drink consumption.[6] Campaign developers may therefore wish to focus countermarketing efforts toward communities considering sugary drink reduction policies so that campaigns can simultaneously support both individual behavior change and policy adoption.

The countermarketing messages elicited more message reactance than the health education messages, which could reduce their ability to change behavior given that reactance is theorized to undermine the beneficial effects of health messages.[31] However, research has found that the benefits of evocative messages for spurring behavior change can outweigh their effects on reactance.[24]

Limitations

This study had several limitations. First, we recruited a convenience sample that differed somewhat from the US population, perhaps in part because we oversampled young adults. However, gender, race, ethnicity, education, and income did not moderate the effect of the messages on intentions. Moreover, previous studies indicate that randomized experiments conducted with convenience samples yield similar results as those conducted with nationally representative samples,[32,33] including when analyzing specific subgroups.[33] Second, participants had only 1 brief exposure to the messages in the context of an online survey. Repeated or longer exposure to the messages could yield larger effects,[34] while exposure in naturalistic settings with more competition for audience attention could yield smaller effects.

Third, we measured self-reported outcomes (e.g., intentions), so effects on behavioral outcomes (e.g., purchases or consumption) remain unknown. A meta-analysis of experiments found that medium-to-large changes in intentions ($d = 0.64$) lead to small-to-medium changes in behavior ($d = 0.41$).[17] In our study, a single exposure to the messages led to small-to-medium changes in intentions, suggesting that these messages could lead to small reductions in sugary drink consumption. Small reductions in sugary drink consumption can have meaningful public health benefits,[35] but additional strategies beyond media campaigns will be needed to address diet-related chronic diseases. Moreover, the success of media campaigns may depend on the resources available to develop and disseminate them; social media may be a promising avenue for dissemination given its relatively low cost per person reached.

Fourth, we did not pretest the messages used in the trial; future studies could refine messages with qualitative or quantitative pretesting to maximize their beneficial effects and minimize unintended consequences. Fifth, it is possible that other features of messages, such as valence or tone, could influence message effectiveness, but we did not test this directly. Sixth, trial messages focused only on discouraging sugary drink consumption, but media campaigns may be even more effective if they also encourage water consumption.[11]

Key strengths of the study include the randomized design, the realistic messages and images that mirrored recent real-world campaigns, and measurement of both intended and unintended consequences.

Conclusions

This randomized trial with a large sample of US adults suggests that countermarketing messages hold promise for reducing sugary drink consumption—especially among young adults—while eliciting less perceived weight stigma than health education messages. Public health departments and nonprofits interested in using media campaigns to reduce sugary drink consumption should consider adopting countermarketing messages in addition to health education messages, though countermarketing messages might need to be refined further to minimize weight stigma and maximize effects on behavior. AJPH

ABOUT THE AUTHORS

Anna H. Grummon is with the Department of Pediatrics and Department of Health Policy, Stanford University School of Medicine, Palo Alto, CA. Amanda B. Zeitlin and Cristina J. Y. Lee are with the Department of Pediatrics, Stanford University School of Medicine. Marissa G. Hall is with the Department of Health Behavior in the University of North Carolina Gillings School of Global Public Health, the Carolina Population Center, and the Lineberger Comprehensive Cancer Center, Chapel Hill. Caroline Collis and Lauren P. Cleveland are with the Department of Population Medicine, Harvard Pilgrim Health Care Institute, Boston, MA. Joshua Petimar is with the Department of Population Medicine, Harvard Medical School and Harvard Pilgrim Health Care Institute, and the Department of Epidemiology, Harvard T.H. Chan School of Public Health, Boston.

CORRESPONDENCE

Correspondence should be sent to Anna H. Grummon, PhD, Stanford University School of Medicine, 3145 Porter Dr, A103, Palo Alto, CA 94304 (e-mail: agrummon@stanford.edu). Reprints can be ordered at https://www.ajph.org by clicking the "Reprints" link.

PUBLICATION INFORMATION

Full Citation: Grummon AH, Zeitlin AB, Lee CJY, et al. Countermarketing versus health education messages about sugar-sweetened beverages: an online randomized controlled trial of US adults. *Am J Public Health*. 2024;114(12):1354–1364.

Acceptance Date: August 16, 2024.

DOI: https://doi.org/10.2105/AJPH.2024.307853

ORCID iDs:

Anna H. Grummon https://orcid.org/0000-0002-8705-038X

Amanda B. Zeitlin https://orcid.org/0009-0005-1822-8198

Cristina J. Y. Lee https://orcid.org/0009-0008-0362-2979

CONTRIBUTORS

A. H. Grummon conceptualized the study, developed the measures, acquired funding, and prepared the original article draft. A. B. Zeitlin contributed to project administration, data analysis, and revising the article. C. J. Y. Lee contributed to data analysis and revising the article. M. G. Hall contributed to conceptualizing the study, developing measures, and revising the article. C. Collis and L. P. Cleveland contributed to project administration and revising the article. J. Petimar contributed to conceptualizing the study, acquiring funding, and revising the article.

ACKNOWLEDGMENTS

This project was funded in part by a grant from the Department of Population Medicine, Harvard Pilgrim Health Care Institute to J. Petimar and A. H. Grummon.

We thank Sara Cathey for graphic design support.

CONFLICTS OF INTEREST

The authors have no conflicts of interest to disclose.

HUMAN PARTICIPANT PROTECTION

The Stanford University (69580) and Harvard Pilgrim Health Care (882) institutional review boards approved the study. We preregistered the study design and statistical analysis plan before data collection on ClinicalTrials.gov (NCT05953194) and AsPredicted.org (https://aspredicted.org/HY8_KVV).

REFERENCES

1. Centers for Disease Control and Prevention. Get the facts: sugar-sweetened beverages and consumption. April 11, 2022. Available at: https://www.cdc.gov/nutrition/data-statistics/sugar-sweetened-beverages-intake.html. Accessed October 6, 2023.
2. Wakefield MA, Loken B, Hornik RC. Use of mass media campaigns to change health behaviour. *Lancet*. 2010;376(9748):1261–1271. https://doi.org/10.1016/S0140-6736(10)60809-4
3. Kraak VI, Consavage Stanley K, Harrigan PB, Zhou M. How have media campaigns been used to promote and discourage healthy and unhealthy beverages in the United States? A systematic scoping review to inform future research to reduce sugary beverage health risks. *Obes Rev*. 2022;23(5):e13425. https://doi.org/10.1111/obr.13425
4. Farley TA, Halper HS, Carlin AM, Emmerson KM, Foster KN, Fertig AR. Mass media campaign to reduce consumption of sugar-sweetened beverages in a rural area of the United States. *Am J Public Health*. 2017;107(6):989–995. https://doi.org/10.2105/AJPH.2017.303750
5. Morley BC, Niven PH, Dixon HG, Swanson MG, McAleese AB, Wakefield MA. Controlled cohort evaluation of the LiveLighter mass media campaign's impact on adults' reported consumption of sugar-sweetened beverages. *BMJ Open*. 2018;8(4):e019574. https://doi.org/10.1136/bmjopen-2017-019574
6. Palmedo PC, Dorfman L, Garza S, Murphy E, Freudenberg N. Countermarketing alcohol and unhealthy food: an effective strategy for preventing noncommunicable diseases? Lessons from tobacco. *Annu Rev Public Health*. 2017;38(1):119–144. https://doi.org/10.1146/annurev-publhealth-031816-044303
7. Harris J, Fleming-Milici F. Food marketing to adolescents and young adults: skeptical but still under the influence. In: Folkvord F, ed. *The Psychology of Food Marketing and Overeating*. London, UK: Routledge; 2019:25–43. https://doi.org/10.4324/9780429274404-3
8. Choi YY, Andreyeva T, Fleming-Milici F, Harris JLUS. Households' children's drink purchases: 2006–2017 trends and associations with marketing. *Am J Prev Med*. 2022;62(1):9–17. https://doi.org/10.1016/j.amepre.2021.06.013
9. Hawaii State Department of Health. Sweet lies. Living Healthy Hawaii. 2023. Available at: https://livinghealthy.hawaii.gov/sweetlies. Accessed March 13, 2024.
10. LaRose JG, Leahey TM, Hill JO, Wing RR. Differences in motivations and weight loss behaviors in young adults and older adults in the National Weight Control Registry. *Obesity (Silver Spring)*. 2013;21(3):449–453. https://doi.org/10.1002/oby.20053
11. Krieger J, Kwon T, Ruiz R, Walkinshaw LP, Yan J, Roberto CA. Countermarketing about fruit drinks, alone or with water promotion: a 2019 randomized controlled trial in Latinx parents. *Am J Public Health*. 2021;111(11):1997–2007. https://doi.org/10.2105/AJPH.2021.306488
12. Harris JL, Phaneuf L, Fleming-Milici F. Effects of sugary drink countermarketing videos on caregivers' attitudes and intentions to serve fruit drinks and toddler milks to young children. *Am J Public Health*. 2022;112(suppl 8):S807–S816. https://doi.org/10.2105/AJPH.2022.307024
13. Bryan CJ, Yeager DS, Hinojosa CP. A values-alignment intervention protects adolescents from the effects of food marketing. *Nat Hum Behav*. 2019;3(6):596–603. https://doi.org/10.1038/s41562-019-0586-6
14. Hayward LE, Vartanian L. Potential unintended consequences of graphic warning labels on sugary drinks: do they promote obesity stigma? *Obes Sci Pract*. 2019;5(4):333–341. https://doi.org/10.1002/osp4.353
15. Puhl RM, Himmelstein MS, Pearl RL. Weight stigma as a psychosocial contributor to obesity. *Am Psychol*. 2020;75(2):274–289. https://doi.org/10.1037/amp0000538
16. Puhl R, Suh Y. Health consequences of weight stigma: implications for obesity prevention and treatment. *Curr Obes Rep*. 2015;4(2):182–190. https://doi.org/10.1007/s13679-015-0153-z
17. McDermott MS, Oliver M, Iverson D, Sharma R. Effective techniques for changing physical activity and healthy eating intentions and behaviour: a systematic review and meta-analysis. *Br J Health Psychol*. 2016;21(4):827–841. https://doi.org/10.1111/bjhp.12199
18. Grummon AH, Brewer NT. Health warnings and beverage purchase behavior: mediators of impact. *Ann Behav Med*. 2020;54(9):691–702. https://doi.org/10.1093/abm/kaaa011
19. Puhl R, Luedicke J, Lee Peterson J. Public reactions to obesity related health campaigns: a randomized controlled trial. *Am J Prev Med*. 2013;45(1):36–48. https://doi.org/10.1016/j.amepre.2013.02.010
20. Donnelly GE, Zatz LY, Svirsky D, John LK. The effect of graphic warnings on sugary-drink purchasing. *Psychol Sci*. 2018;29(8):1321–1333. https://doi.org/10.1177/0956797618766361
21. Nan X, Heo K. Consumer responses to corporate social responsibility (CSR) initiatives: examining the role of brand-cause fit in cause-related marketing. *J Advert*. 2007;36(2):63–74. https://doi.org/10.2753/JOA0091-3367360204
22. Hall MG, Sheeran P, Noar SM, Ribisl KM, Boynton MH, Brewer NT. A brief measure of reactance to health warnings. *J Behav Med*. 2017;40(3):520–529. https://doi.org/10.1007/s10865-016-9821-z
23. Noar SM, Barker J, Bell T, Yzer M. Does perceived message effectiveness predict the actual effectiveness of tobacco education messages? A systematic review and meta-analysis. *Health Commun*. 2020;35(2):148–157. https://doi.org/10.1080/10410236.2018.1547675
24. Hall MG, Sheeran P, Noar SM, et al. Negative affect, message reactance and perceived risk: how do pictorial cigarette pack warnings change quit intentions? *Tob Control*. 2018;27(e2):e136–e142. https://doi.org/10.1136/tobaccocontrol-2017-053972
25. Hong SM, Faedda S. Refinement of the Hong psychological reactance scale. *Educ Psychol Meas*. 1996;56(1):173–182. https://doi.org/10.1177/0013164496056001014
26. Harris KM, Udry JR. National Longitudinal Study of Adolescent to Adult Health (Add Health), 1994–2018 [Public Use]. Chapel Hill, NC: Carolina Population Center, University of North Carolina-Chapel Hill, Inter-university Consortium for

Political and Social Research; 2022. https://doi.org/10.3886/ICPSR21600.v25

27. Cohen J. *Statistical Power Analysis for the Behavioral Sciences.* New York, NY: Academic Press; 2013. https://doi.org/10.4324/9780203771587
28. Dunn JE, Liu K, Greenland P, Hilner JE, Jacobs DR Jr. Seven-year tracking of dietary factors in young adults: the CARDIA study. *Am J Prev Med.* 2000;18(1):38–45. https://doi.org/10.1016/S0749-3797(99)00114-2
29. Holm S. Obesity interventions and ethics. *Obes Rev.* 2007;8(s1):207–210. https://doi.org/10.1111/j.1467-789X.2007.00343.x
30. Ajzen I. Consumer attitudes and behavior. In: Haugtvedt C, Herr P, Cardes F, eds. *Handbook of Consumer Psychology.* New York, NY: Lawrence Erlbaum Associates; 2008:525–548.
31. Brehm SS, Brehm JW. *Psychological Reactance: A Theory of Freedom and Control.* New York, NY: Academic Press; 2013.
32. Jeong M, Zhang D, Morgan J, et al. Similarities and differences in tobacco control research findings from convenience and probability samples. *Ann Behav Med.* 2019;53(5):476–485. https://doi.org/10.1093/abm/kay059
33. Coppock A, Leeper TJ, Mullinix KJ. Generalizability of heterogeneous treatment effect estimates across samples. *Proc Natl Acad Sci USA.* 2018;115(49):12441–12446. https://doi.org/10.1073/pnas.1808083115
34. Schmidt S, Eisend M. Advertising repetition: a meta-analysis on effective frequency in advertising. *J Advert.* 2015;44(4):415–428. https://doi.org/10.1080/00913367.2015.1018460
35. Grummon AH, Smith NR, Golden SD, Frerichs L, Taillie LS, Brewer NT. Health warnings on sugar-sweetened beverages: simulation of impacts on diet and obesity among US adults. *Am J Prev Med.* 2019;57(6):765–774. https://doi.org/10.1016/j.amepre.2019.06.022

The Burden of Injuries Associated With E-Bikes, Powered Scooters, Hoverboards, and Bicycles in the United States: 2019–2022

Kathryn G. Burford, PhD, Nicole G. Itzkowitz, MSc, Andrew G. Rundle, DrPH, Charles DiMaggio, PhD, and Stephen J. Mooney, PhD

Objectives. To describe the national burden of injuries associated with e-bikes, bicycles, hoverboards, and powered scooters (micromobility devices) in the United States.

Methods. We compared patterns and trends for 1 933 296 estimated injuries associated with micromobility devices from 2019 to 2022 using National Electronic Injury Surveillance System data.

Results. The population-based rates of e-bike and powered scooter injuries increased by 293.0% and 88.0%, respectively. When reported, powered scooter injuries had the highest proportion for alcohol use (9.0%) compared with other modes, whereas e-bike injuries had the highest proportion for motor vehicle involvement (35.4%). Internal injuries were more likely among e-bike diagnoses than hoverboard and bicycle ($P < .05$), but fractures and concussions were more likely among hoverboard diagnoses compared with all other devices ($P < .05$). When helmet use was identified in clinical notes (20.3%), helmet usage was higher among e-bike injuries (43.8%) compared with powered scooter (34.8%) and hoverboard (30.3%) injuries but lower compared with bicycle injuries (48.7%).

Conclusions. The incidence of severe e-bike and powered scooter injuries increased over the 4-year period. Public health stakeholders should focus on improved surveillance and prevention of injuries associated with electric micromobility devices. (*Am J Public Health*. 2024;114(12):1365–1374. https://doi.org/10.2105/AJPH.2024.307820)

AJPH December 2024, Vol. 114, No. 12

Micromobility devices, including bicycles, e-bikes, powered scooters, and hoverboards, are gaining popularity as cost-effective, sustainable urban transportation solutions for short-distance travel. While the definition of micromobility is evolving with emerging personal devices and shared systems (e.g., Citi Bike NYC, Lime, Bird), the Federal Highway Administration defines micromobility as "any small, low-speed, human- or electric-powered transportation device."[1]

Micromobility ridership and sales have grown in recent years within the United States.[2,3] Between 2019 and 2022, e-bike sales increased by 269% and surpassed the sales of electric cars and trucks.[3] The number of shared micromobility trips also increased from 64 million trips in 2020 to 112 million in 2021, and, as of 2021, most were by shared electric-powered vehicles (55%, e-scooters; 13%, e-bikes).[4] This surge in micromobility ridership and availability makes it critical to monitor the burden of injuries associated with these transportation modes.

The US Consumer Product Safety Commission released a report in September 2023 using National Electronic Injury Surveillance System (NEISS) data, which showed that from 2017 to 2022, emergency department (ED) visits associated with e-bike and powered scooter usage increased linearly, whereas hoverboard-associated visits decreased during this time.[5] While this report examined several patient and situation characteristics by micromobility device, the authors did not compare the injury type or risk factors for injuries across devices. Understanding how injury types and risk factors vary by mode can inform ED utilization, resource allocation, and intervention strategies and policies to promote safe micromobility use.

Several other studies used NEISS to determine national estimates of injuries related to micromobility devices.[6–13] A study by DiMaggio et al. is the only one of these to describe and compare injury patterns and trends across e-bikes, powered scooters, and pedal bicycles, as most studies focus on only 1 micromobility mode or 1 population (e.g., pediatrics).[7] However, indication of helmet use or alcohol use, 2 risk factors for severe morbidity and mortality in bicycle injury, were not examined.[14,15] Since the study by DiMaggio et al., NEISS also received a major update that improved the reporting of substance use, powered scooters, hoverboards, and additional patient and situation characteristics.[16]

As micromobility availability becomes more widespread in the United States, up-to-date injury surveillance is critical to inform and guide the inconsistent legislation governing micromobility use and to ultimately improve the safety of riders while encouraging usage.[17] This cross-sectional study describes the national burden of injuries associated with micromobility devices by focusing on e-bikes, bicycles, hoverboards, and powered scooters and using 2019–2022 data sourced from NEISS.

METHODS

For this cross-sectional study, we obtained 2019 through 2022 data from the Consumer Product Safety Commission's NEISS query system. NEISS is a nationally representative stratified probability sample of 96 hospitals in the United States and its territories that contain at least 6 beds and an ED.[18] The stratified sample is based on hospital size and geographic location. Each of the 1 331 870 cases from the 2019–2022 NEISS data are assigned a weight to provide nationally representative estimates of injuries that resulted in an ED discharge. Population estimates were obtained from the US Census Bureau for each year of the study.[19]

Data Coding

We generated indicator variables for powered scooter-, e-bike-, and hoverboard-related injuries using product codes and narrative texts (see Appendix Table A [available as a supplement to the online version of this article at https://ajph.org] for a list of product codes and search terms). We included sex, race, ethnicity, location of incident, alcohol use, and drug use as reported within the NEISS coding manual.[16] NEISS only collects positive notations for alcohol use and drug use and, thus, negative notations may be included within the "not reported" categories for each variable. We categorized ages into younger than 5, 5 to 9, 10 to 14, 15 to 17, 18 to 44, 45 to 64, 65 to 84, and older than 84 years, with pediatric age groups considered as aged younger than 18 years. These age groups are consistent with available census data to calculate population-based rates.

To generate a motor vehicle variable, we extracted observations for patient narratives that contained "car," "vehicle," "truck," "bus," or "SUV" terms. For the pedestrian variable, we extracted observations that contained the term "pedestrian."[7] We used the disposition and diagnosis variables as reported within the NEISS coding manual to generate variables for death (dead on arrival, died in the ED, or died after admission), hospitalization (treated and admitted for hospitalization), concussion, internal organ injury, fracture, soft-tissue injury (avulsion, strain, sprain, contusion, abrasion, or laceration), head injury (concussion, internal head injury, external head injury, hematoma, or other head-related injury), and burn (electrical, no specified, scald, chemical, thermal, radiation). A helmet indicator was created using a text-string search approach to extract data from the patient clinical notes, which was operationalized to yes, patient was wearing a helmet; no, patient was not wearing a helmet; or not reported, unknown use of helmet, or no helmet term found within narrative text (code for helmet use and other clinical note–generated variables are available to access in Zenodo).

Analysis

We used statistical weights to generate population estimates. When the patient had more than 1 micromobility mode reported as involved with the injury, we excluded these unweighted records before analysis ($n = 160$). We used the R package "survey" to generate stratified, weighted, nested, year-adjusted survey estimates.[20] Descriptive analyses included total count of injuries that resulted in an ED visit with proportions along with 95% confidence intervals (CIs), which captures the variability based in the NEISS sampling design, stratified by micromobility device. We used survey-adjusted generalized linear models with a log link function (log-binomial regression) to estimate prevalence ratios (PRs) with 95% CIs comparing disposition and diagnoses between micromobility devices. We used US Census Bureau population estimates to calculate injury and age-specific rates per 100 000 population. We performed all analyses using R statistical software (version 4.3.1; R Core Team 2023, Vienna, Austria). Data and code are available to access in Zenodo.

RESULTS

Out of the 48 857 022 (95% CI = 44 571 027, 53 143 018) total injuries that resulted in an ED visit between 2019 and 2022, there were 1 933 296 (95% CI = 1 717 064, 2 149 529) estimated micromobility injuries. Of these micromobility injuries, most involved bicycles (1 623 143; 95% CI = 1 436 665, 1 809 621), accounting for 33.2 (95% CI = 31.3, 35.2) injuries per 1000 total US ED injuries during the 4 years. Over this 4-year time period, there were an estimated 164 712 (95% CI = 132 797, 196 628) powered scooter injuries accounting for 3.4 (95% CI = 2.7, 4.1) injuries per 1000 total ED injuries. There were also an estimated 56 963 (95% CI = 41 206, 72 721) e-bike injuries or 1.2 (95% CI = 0.9, 1.5) injuries per 1000 total ED injuries, and 88 478 (95% CI = 73 882, 103 073) hoverboard injuries, which accounted for 1.8 (95% CI = 1.6, 2.0) injuries per 1000 total ED injuries between 2019 and 2022.

Demographics

Table 1 reports the demographics of individuals injured across micromobility modes. Of all estimated hoverboard injuries, 76.2% (95% CI = 69.7%, 83.6%) were among those aged younger than 18 years compared with 14.5% (95% CI = 10.3%, 20.7%) of e-bike injuries and 16.1% (95% CI = 12.5%, 20.8%) of powered scooter injuries. By contrast, 57.2% (95% CI = 53.2%, 61.1%) of powered scooter injuries, 48.6% (95% CI = 42.8%, 54.4%) of e-bike injuries, and 30.6% (95% CI = 28.2%, 33.1%) of bicycle injuries were among those aged 18 to 44 years, while 16.7% (95% CI = 14.0%, 19.9%) of hoverboard injuries were among those aged 18 to 44 years (Figure 1). Among older adults (65–84 years), the highest proportion of micromobility injuries was bicycle-related (11.8%; 95% CI = 9.7%, 14.3%) and was closely followed by e-bike–related injuries (9.6%; 95% CI = 7.5%, 12.4%). Within the pediatric population (< 18 years), most hoverboard injuries were among those aged 5 to 9 years (41.3%; 95% CI = 38.3%, 44.4%) followed by those aged 10 to 14 years (28.5%; 95% CI = 26.3%, 30.9%).

The proportion of males injured in a powered scooter (63.9%; 95% CI = 60.0%, 67.7%), e-bike (76.9%; 95% CI = 72.9%, 80.5%), and bicycle (73.7%; 95% CI = 72.3%, 75.0%) -related incident was higher compared with females. When patient records included race, the proportions for powered scooter, e-bike, hoverboard, and bicycle injuries were higher among White patients compared with patients of all other reported races, which ranged from 61.2% (95% CI = 53.1%, 68.8%) for powered scooters to 76.0% (95% CI = 72.3%, 79.4%) for bicycles. When ethnicity was reported, the proportion of Hispanic patients was similar for powered scooter (12.7%; 95% CI = 9.9%, 16.1%), e-bike (13.2%; 95% CI = 9.6%, 18.0%), bicycle (11.9%; 95% CI = 9.9%, 14.2%), and hoverboard (12.6%; 95% CI = 9.7%, 16.4%) -associated injuries.

Risk Factors

Most e-bike (80.4%; 95% CI = 73.8%, 85.6%), powered scooter (68.9%; 95% CI = 61.4%, 75.5%), and bicycle (58.3%; 95% CI = 54.8%, 61.8%) injuries were reported as taking place on a street or highway, as compared with most hoverboard injuries taking place on private property (76.1%; 95% CI = 70.7%, 80.8%). When a positive indication was reported, powered scooter injuries had higher proportions for involving alcohol use (9.0%; 95% CI = 7.2%, 11.1%) and pedestrians (1.1%; 95% CI = 0.8%, 1.6%) compared with e-bike (6.5%; 95% CI = 5.0%, 8.4% and 1.0%; 95% CI = 0.5%, 1.9%), bicycle (4.1%; 95% CI = 3.6%, 4.6% and 0.6%; 95% CI = 0.5%, 0.8%), and hoverboard (0.7%; 95% CI = 0.4%, 1.3% and 0.1%; 95% CI = 0.02%, 0.40%) injuries. E-bike injuries had higher proportions of reported drug use (3.2%; 95% CI = 2.3%, 4.4%) and motor vehicle involvement (35.4%; 95% CI = 29.3%, 41.9%) compared with powered scooter (1.8%; 95% CI = 1.4%, 2.4% and 25.4%; 95% CI = 19.6%, 32.1%) and bicycle (1.7%; 95% CI = 1.4%, 2.0% and 21.9%; 95% CI = 20.1%, 23.9%) injuries. When helmet use was identified in clinical notes (20.3%), indication of helmet use was higher among e-bike injuries (43.8%; 95% CI = 37.5%, 50.3%) compared with powered scooter (34.8%; 95% CI = 30.7%, 39.0%) and hoverboard (30.3%; 95% CI = 19.0%, 44.7%) injuries but lower compared with bicycle injuries (48.7%; 95% CI = 45.3%, 52.1%).

Disposition and Diagnoses

In descriptive analyses (Table 2), 12.7% (95% CI = 9.4%, 17.0%) of e-bike–related injuries resulted in hospitalization compared with 10.2% (95% CI = 9.0%, 11.6%) for powered scooters, 10.5% (95% CI = 9.6%, 12.1%) for bicycles, and 3.2% (95% CI = 2.5%, 4.0%)

TABLE 1— Descriptive Characteristics for Micromobility Injuries in the National Electronic Injury Surveillance System: United States, 2019–2022

Characteristic	Bicycle (n = 1 623 143), % (95% CI)	E-Bike (n = 56 963), % (95% CI)	Hoverboard (n = 88 477), % (95% CI)	Powered Scooter (n = 164 712), % (95% CI)
Age, y				
<5	3.4 (3.0, 3.8)	0.7 (0.2, 1.8)	4.3 (3.5, 5.4)	0.8 (0.5, 1.3)
5–9	11.1 (9.9, 12.4)	2.4 (1.6, 3.8)	41.3 (38.3, 44.4)	4.0 (3.0, 5.3)
10–14	14.5 (13.2, 15.9)	6.9 (5.2, 9.1)	28.5 (26.3, 30.9)	7.4 (5.8, 9.4)
15–17	5.0 (4.6, 5.4)	4.5 (3.3, 6.1)	2.1 (1.6, 2.9)	3.9 (3.2, 4.8)
18–44	30.6 (28.2, 33.1)	48.6 (42.8, 54.4)	16.7 (14.0, 19.9)	57.2 (53.2, 61.1)
45–64	23.1 (22.1, 24.2)	27.3 (24.0, 30.8)	5.8 (4.5, 7.5)	19.4 (17.8, 21.2)
65–84	11.8 (9.7, 14.3)	9.6 (7.5, 12.4)	1.1 (0.7, 1.8)	6.2 (4.9, 7.7)
>84	0.5 (0.4, 0.7)	0.06 (0.0, 0.2)	0.0 (<0.01, <0.01)	1.1 (0.7, 1.7)
Not reported	0.04 (0.0, 0.1)	0.0 (<0.01, <0.01)	0.0 (<0.01, <0.01)	0.0 (<0.01, 0.1)
Sex				
Male	73.7 (72.3, 75.0)	76.9 (72.9, 80.5)	44.7 (42.3, 47.1)	63.9 (60.0, 67.6)
Female	26.3 (25.0, 27.6)	23.1 (19.5, 27.1)	55.3 (52.9, 57.7)	36.1 (32.4, 40.0)
Intersex/nonbinary	0.009 (<0.01, 0.03)	0.0 (<0.01, <0.01)	0.0 (<0.01, 0.1)	0.1 (<0.01, 0.3)
Not reported	0.0 (<0.01, <0.01)	0.0 (<0.01, <0.01)	0.0 (<0.01, <0.01)	0.0 (<0.01, <0.01)
Race				
American Indian/Alaska Native	0.7 (0.5, 0.9)	0.4 (0.1, 1.2)	0.6 (0.2, 1.5)	0.6 (0.4, 1.0)
Asian	2.4 (2.0, 3.0)	2.9 (1.8, 4.8)	1.6 (0.9, 2.6)	3.0 (2.1, 4.4)
Black/African American	17.2 (13.7, 21.3)	30.9 (19.4, 45.4)	20.1 (16.6, 24.2)	31.7 (23.3, 41.6)
Native Hawaiian/Pacific Islander	0.2 (0.1, 0.3)	0.1 (0.01, 0.6)	0.4 (0.1, 1.1)	0.2 (0.1, 0.5)
Other	3.5 (2.6, 4.5)	3.0 (1.4, 6.5)	4.3 (2.9, 6.4)	3.1 (2.0, 4.9)
White	76.0 (72.3, 79.4)	62.7 (50.6, 73.4)	73.1 (68.9, 77.0)	61.2 (53.1, 68.8)
Not reported	34.2 (26.3, 43.1)	25.6 (16.7, 37.2)	37.8 (27.6, 49.3)	19.2 (14.5, 25.1)
Ethnicity				
Hispanic	11.9 (9.9, 14.2)	13.2 (9.6, 18.0)	12.6 (9.7, 16.4)	12.7 (9.9, 16.1)
Not Hispanic	88.1 (85.8, 90.1)	86.8 (82.0, 90.4)	87.4 (83.6, 90.3)	87.3 (83.9, 90.1)
Not reported	38.2 (29.6, 47.6)	52.7 (37.4, 67.5)	38.9 (28.6, 50.3)	34.4 (23.0, 47.9)
Location of injury				
Place of recreation or sport	12.8 (10.8, 15.2)	3.6 (2.0, 6.5)	5.1 (3.1, 8.2)	2.4 (1.6, 3.6)
Private property	13.2 (11.4, 15.2)	4.1 (2.4, 6.9)	76.1 (70.7, 80.8)	8.5 (6.3, 11.3)
Public property	15.1 (12.6, 18.0)	11.9 (8.5, 16.3)	6.7 (4.5, 9.9)	20.1 (15.6, 25.5)
School or daycare	0.6 (0.5, 0.7)	0.1 (<0.01, 0.4)	0.2 (0.1, 1.1)	0.2 (0.1, 0.7)
Street or highway	58.3 (54.8, 61.8)	80.4 (73.8, 85.6)	11.9 (7.99, 17.2)	68.9 (61.4, 75.5)
Not reported	41.5 (37.1, 46.0)	31.0 (24.5, 38.3)	50.1 (42.9, 57.2)	36.3 (30.4, 42.6)
Alcohol use				
Yes	4.1 (3.6, 4.6)	6.5 (5.0, 8.4)	0.7 (0.4, 1.3)	9.0 (7.2, 11.1)
Not reported	95.9 (95.4, 96.4)	93.5 (91.6, 95.0)	99.3 (98.7, 99.6)	91.0 (88.9, 92.8)
Drug use				
Yes	1.7 (1.4, 2.0)	3.2 (2.3, 4.4)	0.1 (<0.01, 0.5)	1.8 (1.4, 2.4)
Not reported	98.3 (98.0, 98.6)	96.8 (95.6, 97.7)	99.9 (99.5, 100.0)	98.2 (97.6, 98.6)
Motor vehicle involved				
Yes	21.9 (20.1, 23.9)	35.4 (29.3, 41.9)	3.5 (2.7, 4.7)	25.4 (19.6, 32.1)
Not reported	78.1 (76.1, 79.9)	64.6 (58.1, 70.7)	96.5 (95.3, 97.4)	74.6 (67.9, 80.4)

Continued

TABLE 1— Continued

Characteristic	Bicycle (n = 1 623 143), % (95% CI)	E-Bike (n = 56 963), % (95% CI)	Hoverboard (n = 88 477), % (95% CI)	Powered Scooter (n = 164 712), % (95% CI)
Pedestrian involved				
Yes	0.6 (0.5, 0.8)	1.0 (0.5, 1.9)	0.1 (0.02, 0.40)	1.1 (0.8, 1.6)
Not reported	99.4 (99.2, 99.5)	99.0 (98.1, 99.5)	99.9 (99.6, 100.0)	98.9 (98.4, 99.2)
Helmet use				
Yes	48.7 (45.3, 52.1)	43.8 (37.5, 50.3)	30.3 (19.0, 44.7)	34.8 (30.7, 39.0)
No	51.3 (47.9, 54.7)	56.2 (49.7, 62.5)	69.7 (55.3, 81.0)	65.2 (61.0, 69.3)
Not reported	80.5 (77.9, 82.8)	68.9 (62.7, 74.5)	97.1 (95.9, 97.9)	78.3 (72.9, 82.9)

Note. CI = confidence interval.

for hoverboards. However, analytic analyses revealed that e-bike–related ED visits were only significantly more likely to be severe enough to result in hospitalization (PR = 4.0; 95% CI = 2.8, 5.8) and diagnoses of a soft tissue injury (PR = 1.4; 95% CI = 1.3, 1.5) and head injury (PR = 1.3; 95% CI = 1.1, 1.7) compared with hoverboard-related ED visits. In addition, internal injuries were more likely to be diagnosed among e-bike ED visits compared with hoverboard (PR = 1.7; 95% CI = 1.2, 2.2) and bicycle ED visits (PR = 1.2, 95% CI = 1.01, 1.5). E-bike ED visits were also 5 times more likely to result in a burn diagnosis compared with bicycle ED visits (PR = 5.0; 95% CI = 1.8, 14.3). Lastly, hoverboard ED visits were more likely to result in diagnoses of fractures and concussions compared with e-bike (PR = 1.4; 95% CI = 1.2, 1.6 and PR = 2.8; 95% CI = 1.6, 5.0), powered scooter (PR = 1.3; 95% CI = 1.2, 1.4 and PR = 1.5; 95% CI = 1.0, 2.05), and bicycle ED visits (PR = 1.4; 95% CI = 1.3, 1.5 and PR = 1.3; 95% CI = 1.05, 1.7).

Trends

The population-based rate of e-bike–related injuries increased between 2019 and 2022 by 293.0% (Appendix Figure A, Appendix Table B). This linear relationship was consistent across all age groups (Figure 2), except for among adults aged older than 84 years, for whom rates were vanishingly small and insignificant (Appendix Table C). While the population-based rate of powered scooter injuries increased by 88.0% over the 4-year period, by 2022, the rate of injuries began to plateau (Appendix Figure A, Appendix Table B), with some evidence of a decrease in injuries among the group aged 18 to 44 years in late 2022 (Figure 2, Appendix Table C). The population-based rates of hoverboard and bicycle injuries were highest before 2021 but since then have declined, with hoverboard injury rates decreasing by 26.2% from 2019 to 2022 (Appendix Figure A, Appendix Table B).

DISCUSSION

In this study, we described and compared the burden of injuries associated with e-bikes, bicycles, hoverboards, and powered scooters within the United States during a time of significant advancement for the electric micromobility industry. Overall, the rate of hoverboard-related injuries decreased over the 4 years and among the pediatric population who experienced the greatest burden of these injuries. This may be explained by hoverboards becoming less popular or could be evidence to support pediatric injury-prevention efforts such as the statement released in 2018 by the American Academic of Pediatrics warning of the dangers of hoverboard use.[21] Conversely, the population-based rate of e-bike–related injuries increased by nearly 300% between 2019 and 2022, which closely parallels the increases in e-bike sales and shared e-bike ridership.[3,4] The rate of powered scooter–associated injuries almost doubled, which may be explained by the increase in shared e-scooter trips across the United States.[4] The increase in electric micromobility injuries might also be attributable to the lack of access, education, and regulation for protective equipment as shared micromobility systems are not required to provide helmets to users. The legislation for where to ride these devices or for riding these devices under the influence is also lacking and inconsistent,[17] and this could lead to greater risks to users such as riding in closer proximity to motor vehicles or while intoxicated.

Those seeking ED care for e-bike, powered scooter, and bicycle injuries

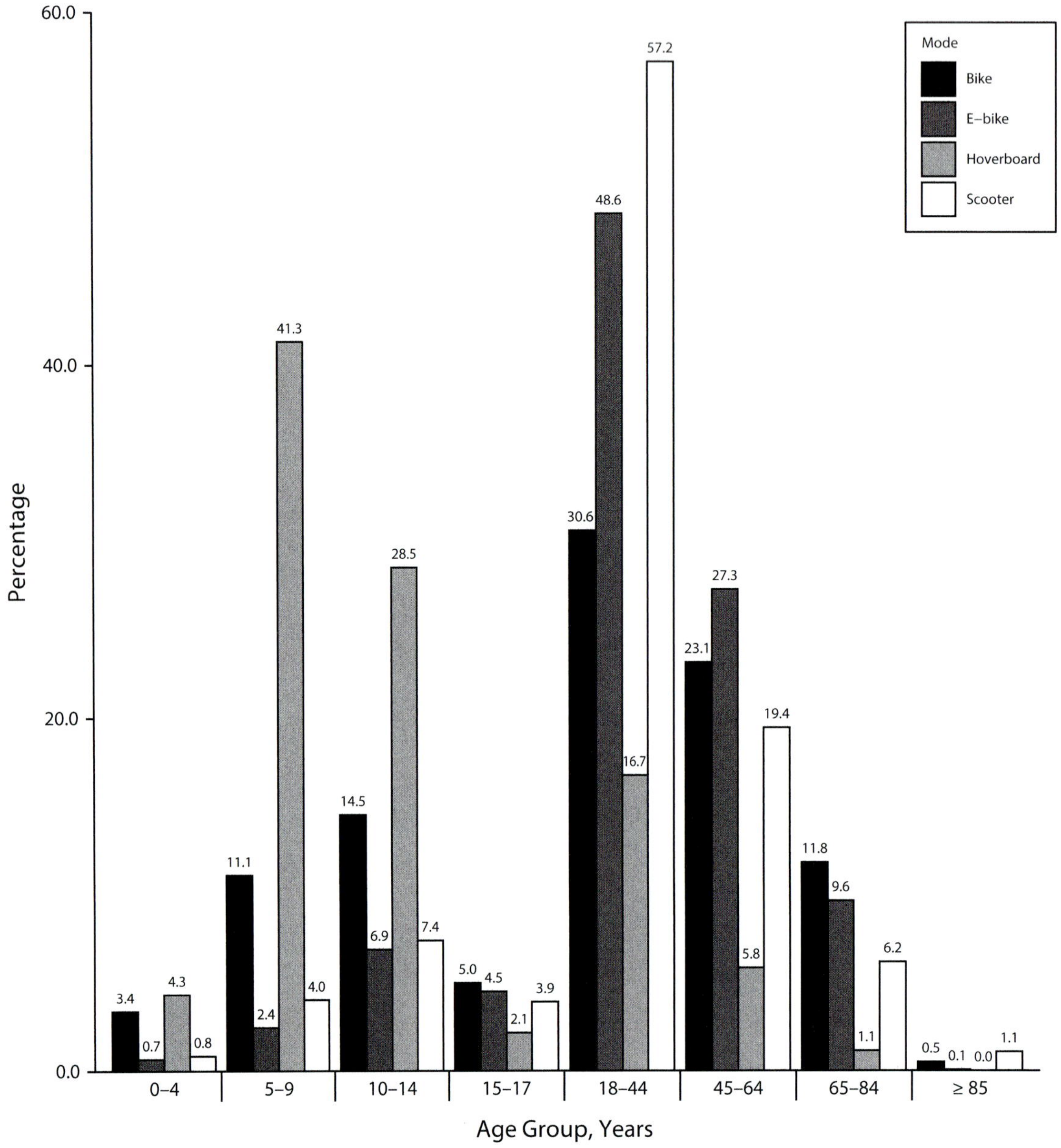

FIGURE 1— **Percentage of Bicycle, E-Bike, Hoverboard, and Powered Scooter Injuries by Age: National Electronic Injury Surveillance System, United States, 2019–2022**

were more often middle-aged, male, and White. One explanation for these findings is that men tend to use e-bikes and e-scooters more than women and engage in riskier behaviors such as alcohol use, which may place them at greater risk of injury.[5,22] Men have also been found to travel faster on e-scooters and to be more likely to use alcohol, drugs, or a smartphone while riding e-scooters compared with women.[23]

In alignment with the Consumer Product Safety Commission's recent report, we found that while the highest proportion of injuries across all micromobility modes was among White patients compared with patients of other races, the proportion of e-bike and powered scooter injuries among Black/African American patients was disproportionately high compared with the percentage of Black Americans in the general population (about 13%).[5,24] However these results should be interpreted with caution because of the incomplete race and ethnicity data, a

TABLE 2— Descriptive Characteristics of Disposition and Diagnoses for Micromobility Injuries in the National Electronic Injury Surveillance System: United States, 2019–2022

Characteristic	Bicycle (n = 1 623 143), % (95% CI)	E-Bike (n = 56 963), % (95% CI)	Hoverboard (n = 88 477), % (95% CI)	Powered Scooter (n = 164 712), % (95% CI)
Disposition				
Died	0.15 (0.1, 0.21)	0.03 (< 0.01, 0.2)	0.00 (< 0.01, < 0.01)	0.14 (0.1, 0.4)
Hospitalized	10.5 (9.6, 12.1)	12.7 (9.4, 17.0)	3.2 (2.5, 4.0)	10.2 (9.0, 11.6)
Diagnoses				
Concussion	3.1 (2.7, 3.4)	1.5 (0.9, 2.5)	4.1 (3.2, 5.3)	2.8 (2.2, 3.6)
Internal	14.0 (13.0, 15.1)	17.4 (13.6, 22.1)	10.5 (8.9, 12.3)	13.9 (12.4, 15.6)
Fractures	29.2 (28.1, 30.5)	29.7 (25.9, 33.8)	41.6 (39.2, 44.1)	31.8 (29.9, 33.7)
Soft tissue	51.5 (50.4, 52.6)	54.7 (51.1, 58.3)	39.8 (37.3, 42.3)	52.9 (50.5, 55.3)
Burns	0.06 (0.0, 0.1)	0.3 (0.1, 0.8)	0.0 (< 0.01, 0.1)	0.13 (0.1, 0.3)
Head injury	18.8 (17.8, 19.7)	21.4 (17.6, 25.7)	15.9 (14.2, 17.7)	19.8 (18.0, 21.6)

Note. CI = confidence interval.

well-known limitation of NEISS and other injury surveillance systems.[25] Given this limitation, smaller studies with access to complete race and ethnicity data could seek to identify vulnerable populations who may rely on certain micromobility devices. In New York City, for instance, approximately 65 000 commercial delivery workers, often referred to as "deliveristas," primarily utilize e-bikes, scooters, and mopeds to complete their deliveries, but their safety and occupational risks have rarely been studied.[26,27]

We also observed that powered scooter–associated injuries exhibited the highest prevalence of alcohol use, followed by e-bike–associated injuries.

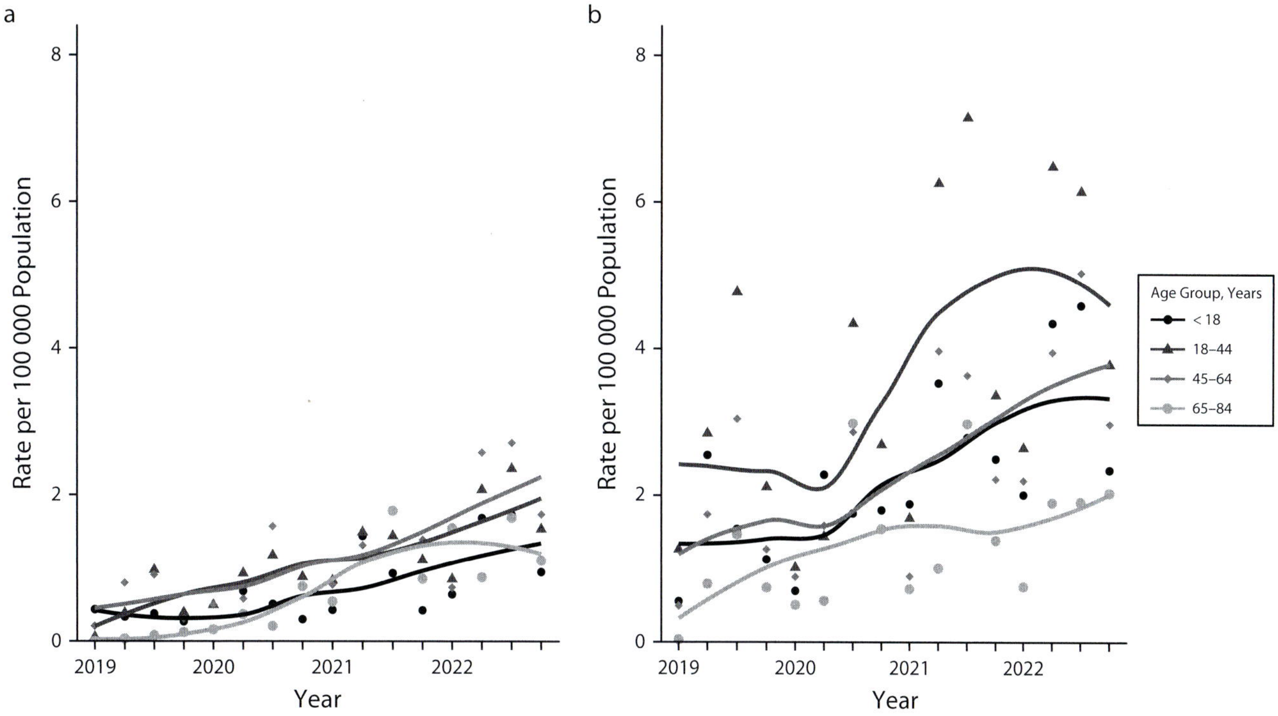

FIGURE 2— Quarterly Rate per 100 000 US Population by Age for (a) E-Bike and (b) Powered Scooter Injuries: National Electronic Injury Surveillance System, 2019–2022

AJPH December 2024, Vol. 114, No. 12

These findings suggest that alcohol involvement may be a public health concern in electric micromobility-related injuries. Yet, again, these results should be interpreted with caution as NEISS only collects data on positive indications of alcohol use and codes a subjective measure of acute alcohol use based on if clinicians' notes mention alcohol involvement. Thus, this existing method for collecting alcohol use likely results in selection bias and measurement error.[28] To improve our understanding of the risk of alcohol use in electric micromobility injuries, future studies are needed that incorporate objective measures of acute alcohol use such as blood alcohol content and more robust epidemiological study designs to determine if alcohol use is a risk factor for these injuries. Micromobility injuries that involve alcohol may be in close proximity to alcohol-serving establishments, nightlife districts, or university or college campuses where micromobility shared systems are typically placed.[4,29] One population-level strategy to prevent injuries associated with these devices may be to focus on improving active transportation infrastructure (e.g., traffic slowing, protected bike lanes, wider sidewalks, docking stations) near high-usage locations such as downtown areas and nightlife districts where alcohol consumption is promoted.

We found that when helmet use was reported, in about 20% of patient narratives, the proportions for bicycle and e-bike injuries involving helmet usage was higher than the proportions for injuries associated with powered scooters or hoverboards. The lowest proportion of helmet use was observed among hoverboard injuries, and these injuries were also more likely to be diagnosed as concussions compared with other modes. These data suggest that concussions in hoverboard injuries remain a particular concern for the pediatric population for whom hoverboard injuries were most prevalent in our study. Policy attention to mandating protective gear use among children riding hoverboards may be needed especially if these devices remain popular. The finding for helmet usage among e-bike injuries was somewhat surprising as bicycle shared systems typically do not provide users with helmets, which is likely for hygiene, cost, and logistical reasons. Given the large percentage of missing helmet-use data, the estimates in our study are likely an inaccurate representation of helmet usage across injuries associated with these devices. Yet, our findings for helmet usage among e-bike injuries was identical to that of a recent report,[13] which reviewed all patient narratives for indication of helmet use in the NEISS data set between 2017 and 2022. In addition, a recent study examining the utility and reliability of a large language model and the text-string search approach we used for extracting helmet status from clinical notes showed that the text-string search approach had high validity when compared with a human-coded gold standard.[30] Complete and accurate data for characterizing helmet usage and other risk factors among micromobility users is critical for informing targeted intervention strategies and policies. As mandatory helmet laws are controversial and likely difficult to pass,[31] public health experts could focus attention on helmet use interventions or understanding the safety effects of active transportation infrastructure to prevent micromobility injuries.

In this study, we also found that internal injuries were more likely to be diagnosed in e-bike–related ED visits compared with visits associated hoverboards and bicycles. In addition, burns were more likely to be diagnosed in e-bike ED visits compared with bicycle ED visits. DiMaggio et al. similarly found that e-bike injuries had higher proportions for internal injuries compared with bicyclist and powered scooter injuries, but soft tissue injury proportions were much lower among e-bike ED visits than results in our study.[7] Differences in our findings may ultimately be attributable to the rise in e-bike injuries in recent years. However, evidence is growing to suggest that e-bike injuries are more severe and injure more body parts compared with bicycle injuries,[32] which may reflect the increased speed of travel and weight of e-bikes compared with other micromobility modes.[33] While we found very few burn diagnoses within our study, the highest proportion estimates were for burns were among e-bike–associated ED visits, and there were few burn diagnoses for e-bike injuries overall, which was surprising given the media attention to deadly and injurious fires from lithium-ion batteries used by these devices.[34]

Limitations

This study added to the very little existing knowledge base on important sociodemographic and risk factor variables that might be contributing to micromobility vehicle–related injuries. This gap in the literature is likely because existing national public-use data sets such as NEISS have only recently begun to collect data on electric micromobility devices. While this study improved our limited understanding of the burden of injuries for users of micromobility devices, there are limitations to be noted. First, several estimates for variables across micromobility modes were small (e.g., death, burns) and may be unstable or unreliable. This is an inherent limitation of the NEISS sampling method and, thus, nationally representative studies that do not rely on a probability sample.[18] Ideally, data that provide information on exposure before injury would allow for stronger epidemiological study designs that inform on the risks associated with these micromobility modes. This may ultimately require building partnerships with rideshare systems, emerging crowdsource data, or collecting retrospective data from injured users of these devices.

As previously discussed, measurement error is also a limitation within our study, particularly for variables that were generated exclusively through narrative text (e.g., motor vehicle- or pedestrian-involved, helmet use). Natural language processing or large language models applied to clinical notes could supplement the validated text string approach we developed for helmet status coding to improve its efficiency.[28,35] Overall, while emerging micromobility devices have the potential to provide population-level health, climate, and transportation benefits, implementing uniform definitions of micromobility devices and improving the collection of complete risk factor data within injury surveillance is urgently needed to accurately inform micromobility policies and interventions.

Public Health Implications

In summary, this study highlights numerous public health concerns associated with the burgeoning micromobility industry. While less prevalent than traditional bicycle injuries, the rate of e-bike injuries increased fourfold over the 4-year period, and the rate of powered scooter injuries nearly doubled. Given the ongoing growth of the electric micromobility sector and recent historic investments in active transportation by the federal government, it is imperative for the public health community to advance surveillance and prevention of micromobility-related injuries. AJPH

ABOUT THE AUTHORS

Kathryn G. Burford is with the Department of Environmental Health Sciences, Mailman School of Public Health, Columbia University, New York, NY. Nicole G. Itzkowitz and Andrew G. Rundle are with the Department of Epidemiology, Mailman School of Public Health, Columbia University. Charles DiMaggio is with the Department of Surgery, NYU Grossman School of Medicine, New York, NY. Stephen J. Mooney is with the Department of Epidemiology, School of Public Health, University of Washington, Seattle.

CORRESPONDENCE

Correspondence should be sent to Kathryn G. Burford, Mailman School of Public Health, Columbia University, 722 W 168th St, Room 1616, New York, NY 10031 (e-mail: kb3424@cumc.columbia.edu). Reprints can be ordered at https://www.ajph.org by clicking the "Reprints" link.

PUBLICATION INFORMATION

Full Citation: Burford KG, Itzkowitz NG, Rundle AG, DiMaggio C, Mooney SJ. The burden of injuries associated with e-bikes, powered scooters, hoverboards, and bicycles in the United States: 2019–2022. *Am J Public Health*. 2024;114(12):1365–1374.

Acceptance Date: July 21, 2024.

DOI: https://doi.org/10.2105/AJPH.2024.307820

ORCID iDs:

Kathryn G. Burford https://orcid.org/0000-0001-5500-9609

Nicole G. Itzkowitz https://orcid.org/0000-0001-5076-3522

Andrew G. Rundle https://orcid.org/0000-0003-0211-7707

Charles DiMaggio https://orcid.org/0000-0003-2356-6659

CONTRIBUTORS

K. G. Burford acquired the data, conducted data analyses, and led the writing of the article. All authors conceptualized the study, interpreted results, contributed to the writing of the article, and read and approved the final article.

ACKNOWLEDGMENTS

K. G. Burford and N. G. Itzkowitz are funded by the National Institute of Environmental Health Sciences (KGB: 5T32ES007322-21; NGI: 5T32ES007322-22). A. G. Rundle is supported by Centers for Disease Control and Prevention–funded "The Columbia Center for Injury Science and Prevention" (R49CE003094).

CONFLICTS OF INTEREST

The authors have no conflicts of interest to disclose.

HUMAN PARTICIPANT PROTECTION

The study was exempt from institutional review board approval because this study used publicly available, de-identified data.

REFERENCES

1. Price J, Blackshear D, Blount W Jr, Sandt L. Micromobility: a travel mode innovation. *Public Roads*. 2021;85(1). Publication no. FHWA-HRT-21-003. Available at: https://highways.dot.gov/public-roads/spring-2021/02. Accessed February 5, 2024.
2. Heineke K, Kloss B, Scurtu D. The future of micromobility: Ridership and revenue after a crisis. McKinsey & Company. July 16, 2020. Available at: https://www.mckinsey.com/industries/automotive-and-assembly/our-insights/the-future-of-micromobility-ridership-and-revenue-after-a-crisis. Accessed November 26, 2023.
3. Coren MJ. Think you need another car? Consider an e-bike instead. *Washington Post*. October 17, 2023. Available at: https://www.washingtonpost.com/climate-environment/2023/10/17/electric-bikes-cars-cost-testing. Accessed December 1, 2023.
4. National Association of City Transportation Officials. Shared micromobility in the US 2020–2021. 2022. Available at: https://nacto.org/shared-micromobility-2020-2021. Accessed November 26, 2023.
5. Tark J. *Micromobility Products-Related Deaths, Injuries, and Hazard Patterns: 2017–2022*. Bethesda, MD: US Consumer Product Safety Commission; 2023.
6. Aizpuru M, Farley KX, Rojas JC, Crawford RS, Moore TJ, Wagner ER. Motorized scooter injuries in the era of scooter-shares: a review of the National Electronic Surveillance System. *Am J Emerg Med*. 2019;37(6):1133–1138. https://doi.org/10.1016/j.ajem.2019.03.049
7. DiMaggio CJ, Bukur M, Wall SP, Frangos SG, Wen AY. Injuries associated with electric-powered bikes and scooters: analysis of US consumer product data. *Inj Prev*. 2020;26(6):524–528. https://doi.org/10.1136/injuryprev-2019-043418
8. Farley KX, Aizpuru M, Wilson JM, et al. Estimated incidence of electric scooter injuries in the US from 2014 to 2019. *JAMA Netw Open*. 2020;3(8):e2014500. https://doi.org/10.1001/jamanetworkopen.2020.14500

9. Goodman LF, Birnbaum Flyer Z, Schomberg J, et al. Electric bicycles (e-bikes) are an increasingly common pediatric public health problem. *Surg Open Sci*. 2023;14:46–51. https://doi.org/10.1016/j.sopen.2023.06.004

10. McIlvain C, Hadiza G, Tzavaras TJ, Weingart GS. Injuries associated with hoverboard use: a review of the National Electronic Injury Surveillance System. *Am J Emerg Med*. 2019;37(3):472–477. https://doi.org/10.1016/j.ajem.2018.06.022

11. Namiri NK, Lui H, Tangney T, Allen IE, Cohen AJ, Breyer BN. Electric scooter injuries and hospital admissions in the United States, 2014–2018. *JAMA Surg*. 2020;155(4):357–359. https://doi.org/10.1001/jamasurg.2019.5423

12. Neuroth LM, Humphries KD, Wing JJ, Smith GA, Zhu M. Motor vehicle-related electric scooter injuries in the US: a descriptive analysis of NEISS data. *Am J Emerg Med*. 2022;55:1–5. https://doi.org/10.1016/j.ajem.2022.02.004

13. Fernandez AM, Li KD, Patel HV, et al. Electric bicycle injuries and hospitalizations. *JAMA Surg*. 2024;159(5):586–588. https://doi.org/10.1001/jamasurg.2023.7860

14. Olivier J, Creighton P. Bicycle injuries and helmet use: a systematic review and meta-analysis. *Int J Epidemiol*. 2017;46(1):278–292. https://doi.org/10.1093/ije/dyw153

15. Airaksinen NK, Nurmi-Lüthje IS, Kataja JM, Kröger HPJ, Lüthje PMJ. Cycling injuries and alcohol. *Injury*. 2018;49(5):945–952. https://doi.org/10.1016/j.injury.2018.03.002

16. Consumer Product Safety Commission. *NEISS Coding Manual*. January 2020. Available at: https://www.cpsc.gov/s3fs-public/2020-CPSC-Only-Non-Trauma-Coding-Manual.pdf. Accessed November 26, 2023.

17. Pimentel D, Koglin T, Lowry M. Taming and tapping the bikeshare explosion. Seattle, WA: Pacific Northwest Transportation Consortium; 2020.

18. US Consumer Product Safety Commission. *The National Electronic Injury Surveillance System: A Tool for Researchers*. 2000. Available at: https://www.cpsc.gov/s3fs-public/pdfs/blk_media_2000d015.pdf. Accessed July 16, 2024.

19. US Census Bureau. Age and sex tables. Available at: https://www.census.gov/topics/population/age-and-sex/data/tables.2019.List_897222059.html#list-tab-List_897222059. Accessed November 26, 2023.

20. Lumley T, Gao P, Schneider B. Package 'survey.' May 3, 2023. Available at: https://cran.r-project.org/web/packages/survey/survey.pdf. Accessed November 26, 2023.

21. Korioth T. Hoverboard injuries send thousands of kids to emergency rooms. American Academy of Pediatrics. 2018. Available at: https://publications.aap.org/aapnews/news/11010/Hoverboard-injuries-send-thousands-of-kids-to. Accessed December 3, 2023.

22. Pawlowski B, Atwal R, Dunbar RIM. Sex differences in everyday risk-taking behavior in humans. *Evol Psychol*. 2008;6(1):147470490800600. https://doi.org/10.1177/147470490800600104

23. Gioldasis C, Christoforou Z, Seidowsky R. Risk-taking behaviors of e-scooter users: a survey in Paris. *Accid Anal Prev*. 2021;163:106427. https://doi.org/10.1016/j.aap.2021.106427

24. US Census Bureau. QuickFacts. Available at: https://www.census.gov/quickfacts/fact/table/US/PST045222. Accessed December 3, 2023.

25. Min J, Gurka KK, Kalesan B, Bian J, Prosperi M. Injury burden in the United States: accurate, reliable, and timely surveillance using electronic health care data. *Am J Public Health*. 2019;109(12):1702–1706. https://doi.org/10.2105/AJPH.2019.305306

26. City of New York. Mayor Adams, Majority Leader Schumer announce first-in-nation street deliveristas hubs to serve NYC's food delivery workers. October 3, 2022. Available at: https://www.nyc.gov/office-of-the-mayor/news/715-22/mayor-adams-majority-leader-schumer-first-in-nation-street-deliveristas-hubs-serve#/0. Accessed December 13, 2023.

27. Heyer JH, Sethi M, Wall SP, et al. Drawing the curtain back on injured commercial bicyclists. *Am J Public Health*. 2015;105(10):2131–2136. https://doi.org/10.2105/AJPH.2015.302738

28. Burford KG, Rundle AG, Frangos S, et al. Comparing alcohol involvement among injured pedalcycle and motorcycle riders across three national public-use datasets. *Traffic Inj Prev*. 2024;1–8. https://doi.org/10.1080/15389588.2024.2364358

29. Banerjee S. Kabir MM, Khadem NK, Chavis C. Optimal locations for bikeshare stations: a new GIS based spatial approach. *Transp Res Interdiscip Perspect*. 2020;4:100101. https://doi.org/10.1016/j.trip.2020.100101

30. Burford KG, Itzkowitz NG, Ortega AG, Teitler JO, Rundle AG. Identification of helmet status among patients with micromobility accidents using ChatGPT-4 to analyze unstructured clinical notes. *JAMA Netw Open*. 2024;7(8):e2425981. https://doi.org/10.1001/jamanetworkopen.2024.25981

31. Bachynski K, Bateman-House A. Mandatory bicycle helmet laws in the United States: origins, context, and controversies. *Am J Public Health*. 2020;110(8):1198–1204. https://doi.org/10.2105/AJPH.2020.305718

32. Berk T, Halvachizadeh S, Backup J, et al. Increased injury severity and hospitalization rates following crashes with e-bikes versus conventional bicycles: an observational cohort study from a regional level II trauma center in Switzerland. *Patient Saf Surg*. 2022;16(1):11. https://doi.org/10.1186/s13037-022-00318-9

33. Hu L, Hu X, Wang J, Kuang A, Hao W, Lin M. Casualty risk of e-bike rider struck by passenger vehicle using China in-depth accident data. *Traffic Inj Prev*. 2020;21(4):283–287. https://doi.org/10.1080/15389588.2020.1747614

34. Hu W. How New York plans to regulate e-bikes in the wake of deadly fires. *New York Times*. September 15, 2023. Available at: https://www.nytimes.com/article/ebike-laws-nyc.html. Accessed December 3, 2023.

35. Zhou W, Prater LC, Goldstein EV, Mooney SJ. Identifying rare circumstances preceding female firearm suicides: validating a large language model approach. *JMIR Ment Health*. 2023;10:e49359. https://doi.org/10.2196/49359

Assessment of Health Disparities and Sexual Orientation Response Choices Used in Two US National Population-Based Health Surveys, 2020–2021

Nicole F. Kahn, PhD, MEd, Carolyn T. Halpern, PhD, Dana R. Burshell, MPH, Stephanie M. Hernandez, PhD, and Kerith J. Conron, ScD, MPH

Objectives. To (1) compare responses to 2 survey questions designed to measure sexual orientation and (2) understand how variation in responses is associated with mental health.

Methods. Data were from the National Longitudinal Study of Adolescent to Adult Health (Add Health) Sexual Orientation/Gender Identity, Socioeconomic Status, and Health Across the Life Course (SOGI-SES) study (2020–2021) in the United States. We used the adjusted Wald test to compare proportions of respondents who were (1) categorized as heterosexual or straight and sexual minorities using the sexual orientation questions designed for the Add Health study and the National Health Interview Survey (NHIS) and (2) diagnosed with depression or anxiety or panic disorder.

Results. The Add Health question detected more than twice as many sexual minority respondents as the NHIS question. Those who responded as sexual minorities to the Add Health question but as heterosexual or straight to the NHIS question, primarily "mostly heterosexuals," had mental health outcomes that were more like those who were consistently classified as sexual minorities versus those consistently classified as heterosexual or straight.

Conclusions. Current measures of sexual orientation in national-level surveys may underestimate the sexual minority population and sexual orientation–related health disparities.

Public Health Implications. Results illustrate the need for further research to expand measurement of sexual orientation on population-based health surveys. (*Am J Public Health*. 2024;114(12):1375–1383. https://doi.org/10.2105/AJPH.2024.307839)

AJPH December 2024, Vol. 114, No. 12

The lesbian, gay, bisexual, and transgender (LGBT) population continues to grow, with recent estimates suggesting that LGBT people represent 7.2% of the US adult population.[1] This proportion is even greater among younger generations, with 19.7% of Generation Z (born 1997–2004) and 11.2% of millennials (born 1981–1996) identifying as LGBT compared with 3.3% among Generation X (born 1965–1980).[1] However, these figures vary across surveys,[2] reflecting, at least in part, differences in measurement approaches and specific measures used to identify LGBT people (e.g., measuring both sexual orientation and gender identity with 1 question, different response options).[3]

Sexual orientation is a multidimensional construct that includes aspects of sexual identity, attraction, and behavior, making it particularly difficult to measure comprehensively.[3] Most measurement efforts, including those recommended by the recent report from the National Academies of Sciences, Engineering, and Medicine (NASEM), have focused on the identity dimension of sexual orientation, which is often considered the most relevant for understanding and responding to health disparities and inequities.[4] This is important because lesbian, gay, and bisexual (LGB) populations have been shown to experience significantly poorer health outcomes relative to non-LGB people, particularly related to mental health, which are often attributed to minority stress resulting from stigma, discrimination, and inequitable treatment.[3,5–8]

However, research also shows that some people who report same-sex attraction or behavior do not identify as lesbian, gay, bisexual, or another minority sexual orientation when asked about sexual orientation identity.[9,10] These studies further indicate that those who do not identify with traditional labels such as gay, lesbian, or bisexual may represent an "invisible" sexual minority population that experiences health outcomes that are more similar to other sexual minorities yet are missed by programs and policies intended to address these disparities.[1,3,5,11–13] For example, one study using data from the National Longitudinal Study of Adolescent to Adult Health (Add Health) found that those who characterized their sexual orientation as "mostly heterosexual" comprised the largest sexual minority group among both males and females.[14] Furthermore, levels of perceived stress and depressive symptoms of mostly heterosexual respondents were more similar to those of other sexual minority groups than they were to those of 100% heterosexual respondents.[14] As a result, more research focused on understanding who is detected through various measures of sexual orientation may help not only to identify those who could benefit from targeted services and supports but also to inform efforts to measure sexual orientation in population health surveys.

Thus, based on the NASEM report's recommendation to further improve the quality and inclusivity of current sexual orientation identity measures, the purpose of this study was to (1) describe and compare responses from respondents asked to complete 2 different survey questions designed to measure sexual orientation and (2) understand how variation in responses to these questions are associated with mental health outcomes. We hypothesized that (1) the sexual orientation question that measured sexuality by approximating a continuum would detect more sexual minority respondents compared with the item that uses a narrower set of specific sexual orientation identity labels, and (2) sexual minorities who were undetected by either question (i.e., only identify as heterosexual or straight on 1 of the 2 questions) would exhibit similar mental health outcomes compared with those who were categorized as sexual minorities on both measures.

METHODS

The National Longitudinal Study of Adolescent to Adult Health (Add Health) is a large, nationally representative sample of more than 20 745 in-school adolescents who were in the 7th through 12th grades during the 1994–1995 school year (wave I).[15] The cohort has been followed longitudinally, with wave V completed in 2016–2019 (n = 12 300, ages 33–44 years), and wave VI currently in the field. The Sexual Orientation/Gender Identity, Socioeconomic Status, and Health Across the Life Course (SOGI-SES) study is an ancillary, online survey fielded in the fall of 2020 and spring of 2021.[16] The sampling frame included all living Add Health wave V respondents. Those who identified as mostly heterosexual, bisexual, mostly homosexual, or homosexual; reported same-sex partners at waves III, IV, or V (see Measures); or were discordant on sex assigned at birth and gender expression (e.g., androgynous or gender nonconforming) at wave V were all solicited for participation in SOGI-SES. We refer to these respondents as sexual and gender minorities (SGMs).

The study also included a comparison sample of 1500 non-SGM Add Health respondents who identified as completely heterosexual; did not report same-sex partners at waves III, IV, or V; and were conforming in their gender expression. SGMs were selected with certainty. To obtain the comparison sample, remaining non-SGMs were selected across 16 strata defined by sex assigned at birth, race/ethnicity, and percentage of the federal poverty level (according to the US Census) at wave V to achieve a comparison sample that was diverse across race/ethnicity and economic status and was comparable to the SGM population on proportion female sex assigned at birth.[16] In total, 4661 wave V respondents were selected to participate in the SOGI-SES survey. The final sample included 2614 respondents aged 37 to 46 years—56.5% of the selected sample. We conducted nonbias analyses, and determined relative bias to be moderately small.[13] Thus, weighted estimates from the SOGI-SES study are representative of wave V respondents who were in school and in the 7th through 12th grades in 1994 to 1995.

Measures

Sexual orientation. As a part of the SOGI-SES survey, all respondents were asked 2 survey questions that measured sexual orientation.

One of these items was the Add Health question, which has been asked of all Add Health respondents from wave III in 2001 on and defines sexuality approximating a continuum:

"Please choose the description that best fits how you think about yourself."

- 100% heterosexual (straight)
- Mostly heterosexual (straight), but somewhat attracted to people of your own sex
- Bisexual, that is, attracted to men and women equally
- Mostly homosexual (gay), but somewhat attracted to people of the opposite sex
- 100% homosexual (gay)
- Not sexually attracted to either males or females

The other item was the National Health Interview Survey (NHIS) question, which was developed at the National Center for Health Statistics[17] to measure sexual orientation identity and has been used on the NHIS since 2013.[18] This question was modified slightly by the SOGI-SES investigators, including adding the term bisexual to define what is not straight and adding the last 2 response options to the question.

"Which of the following best represents how you think of yourself?"

- Gay or lesbian
- Straight, that is, not gay, lesbian, or bisexual
- Bisexual
- Something else
- I am not sure of my sexuality (I am "questioning" my sexuality)
- I am not sure what this question is asking

Each respondent received both questions sequentially, but the order in which these 2 items were presented was randomized so that half of respondents received the Add Health question first and vice versa.

Two additional variables, "Undetected by Add Health" and "Undetected by NHIS," were created to categorize those respondents who may have self-identified as a sexual minority on only 1 of the items (see Figure 1 for visual representation of these categories). For the purposes of this article, those who selected "I am not sure what this question is asking" to the NHIS question ($n < 20$) were excluded from the constructed variable and related analyses.

Respondents were included in the "heterosexual or straight" category for each question if they selected "100% heterosexual (straight)" for the Add Health question and "Straight, that is, not gay, lesbian, or bisexual" for the NHIS question. Respondents were included in the "Sexual minority" category if they selected any other response besides heterosexual or straight for both questions. For the Add Health question, the "Undetected sexual minority" category included those who selected "100% heterosexual (straight)" for the Add Health question but a sexual minority response option for the NHIS question. Similarly, the "Undetected sexual minority" category for the NHIS question included those who selected "Straight, that is, not gay, lesbian, or bisexual" for the NHIS question but a sexual minority response option for the Add Health question.

Mental health. Respondents were asked, "Has a doctor, nurse, or other health care provider ever told you that you have or had any of the following?" and given a series of health conditions from which they could select "Yes" or "No." This analysis included lifetime diagnoses of depression and anxiety or panic disorder.

Covariates. Given significant differences in the proportion of men and women who identify as LGB,[1] analyses were completed separately by gender. Sex assigned at birth was measured using an item that asked, "What sex were you assigned at birth, on your original birth certificate?" Response choices were "male" and "female." Gender identity was measured using the following item:

"What is your current gender identity? Select all that apply."

- Male
- Female
- Transgender
- Gender nonbinary/genderqueer
- I am not sure of my gender identity (I am "questioning" my gender identity)
- I do not know what this question is asking [coded as missing]

These 2 items were used to construct the gender variable. We included respondents in the "cisgender male" category if they selected "male" for sex assigned at birth and selected only "male" for gender identity. Similarly, we included respondents in the "cisgender female" category if they selected "female" for sex assigned at birth and selected only "female" for gender identity. We excluded those whose sex assigned at birth did not align with their gender identity or selected more than 1 gender identity from this analysis ($n < 35$) because there were too few transgender respondents to provide group-specific results about sexual orientation response patterns.

Analyses

We used descriptive statistics (frequencies and percentages) to present responses to the Add Health and NHIS questions and the lifetime mental

Undetected by Add Health					
Add Health response	NHIS response				
	Straight	Gay/lesbian	Bisexual	Something else	Questioning
100% heterosexual	Heterosexual/ straight	*Undetected SM*	*Undetected SM*	*Undetected SM*	*Undetected SM*
Mostly heterosexual	SM	SM	SM	SM	SM
Bisexual	SM	SM	SM	SM	SM
Mostly homosexual	SM	SM	SM	SM	SM
100% homosexual	SM	SM	SM	SM	SM
Not attracted to males or females	SM	SM	SM	SM	SM
Undetected by NHIS					
Add Health response	NHIS response				
	Straight	Gay/lesbian	Bisexual	Something else	Questioning
100% heterosexual	Heterosexual/ straight	SM	SM	SM	SM
Mostly heterosexual	*Undetected SM*	SM	SM	SM	SM
Bisexual	*Undetected SM*	SM	SM	SM	SM
Mostly homosexual	*Undetected SM*	SM	SM	SM	SM
100% homosexual	*Undetected SM*	SM	SM	SM	SM
Not attracted to males or females	*Undetected SM*	SM	SM	SM	SM

FIGURE 1— Categorization of Two Sexual Orientation Question Responses From the Sexual Orientation/Gender Identity, Socioeconomic Status, and Health Across the Life Course (SOGI-SES) Study: United States, 2020–2021

Note. Add Health = National Longitudinal Study of Adolescent to Adult Health; NHIS = National Health Interview Study; SM = sexual minority.

health diagnosis variables. Next, we used the adjusted Wald test to compare the proportions of respondents who (1) were categorized as undetected sexual minorities and (2) had ever been diagnosed with depression or anxiety or panic disorder by these sexual orientation categories and by gender. We used the Bonferroni correction to adjust for multiple comparisons, with the *P* level set to .05.

All SOGI-SES respondents have valid sampling weights. We restricted statistical analyses to those respondents who had complete data on all variables of interest (< 5% missing). For all analyses, we used sampling weights and adjusted variance estimates for the Add Health complex survey design to yield population representative estimates and completed them with Stata version 17.0 (StataCorp, College Station, TX).

RESULTS

Of 2576 respondents with complete data on the sexual orientation, sex, and gender items, 50.2% were cisgender males, and 49.8% were cisgender females. The mean age was 40.8 years (SD = 1.9; range = 37–46). A larger proportion of cisgender male (93.9%) and cisgender female respondents (91.2%) identified as "straight" in response to the NHIS question compared with cisgender males (92.2%) and cisgender females (79.1%) who identified as "100% heterosexual" in response to the Add Health question. For both questions, a larger proportion of cisgender females identified as sexual minorities compared with cisgender males.

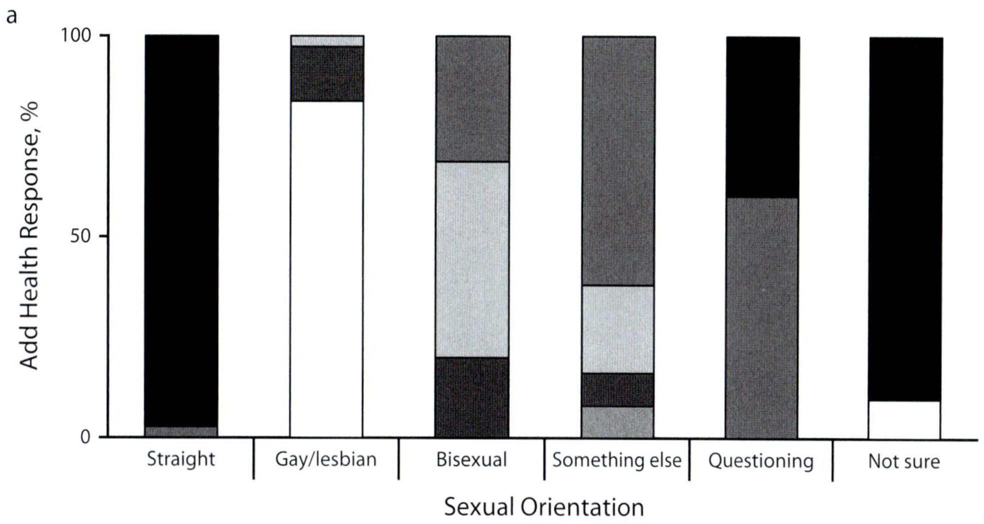

		Straight	Gay/lesbian	Bisexual	Something else	Questioning	Not sure	Total
NHIS response, %		93.9	3.2	1.3	0.6	0.1	0.8	100.0
Add Health response, %								
100% heterosexual		97.3	. . .	. . .	. . .	39.8	90.3	92.2
Mostly heterosexual		2.7	. . .	31.2	62.0	60.2	. . .	3.4
Bisexual		. . .	2.7	48.9	21.9	. . .	. . .	0.9
Mostly homosexual		. . .	13.6	19.9	8.1	. . .	. . .	0.8
100% homosexual		. . .	83.7	. . .	. . .	. . .	9.7	2.8
Not attracted to males or females		< 0.1	. . .	. . .	8.0	. . .	. . .	0.6

FIGURE 2— Sexual Orientation/Gender Identity, Socioeconomic Status, and Health Across the Life Course (SOGI-SES) Study Responses to Two Different Sexual Orientation Questions by (a) Cisgender Male and (b) Cisgender Female: United States, 2020–2021

Note. Add Health = National Longitudinal Study of Adolescent to Adult Health; NHIS = National Health Interview Study. Percentages are weighted to yield population-representative estimates and may not sum to 100% because of rounding.

Comparisons are illustrated in Figure 2 for cisgender males and cisgender females. The vertical bars show how a given Add Health answer maps onto answers to the NHIS question. For example, of the 3.2% of cisgender males who selected "gay/lesbian" for the NHIS question, 2.7% selected "bisexual" in response to the Add Health question, 13.6% selected "mostly homosexual," and 83.7% selected "100% homosexual."

Table 1 shows the proportions of respondents in the combined sexual orientation category variables. For both questions, 85.6% were identified as heterosexual or straight. The Add Health question detected more than twice as many sexual minorities as the NHIS question (14.4% vs 6.8%). Less than 0.1% of respondents were undetected by the Add Health question, while 7.6% of respondents were undetected by the NHIS question. These proportions did not differ by the order in which the questions were asked (Add Health first vs NHIS first; NHIS: $\chi^2 = 0.34$; $P = .66$; Add Health: $\chi^2 = 0.18$; $P = .77$). Nearly all (97.8%) of those undetected by NHIS had responded as "mostly heterosexual" to the Add Health question. Cisgender female respondents were significantly more likely than cisgender male respondents to be undetected by NHIS (12.8% vs 2.6%; $F = 38.73$; $P < .001$). There were no statistically significant differences between cisgender males and cisgender females for the Add Health question (< 0.1% vs < 0.1%; $F = 0.16$; $P = .69$). Given the extremely small number of undetected sexual minorities by the Add Health question, additional analyses could only be completed for the NHIS question.

Results of the mental health diagnosis analyses for the undetected by NHIS variable are shown in Table 2. Overall,

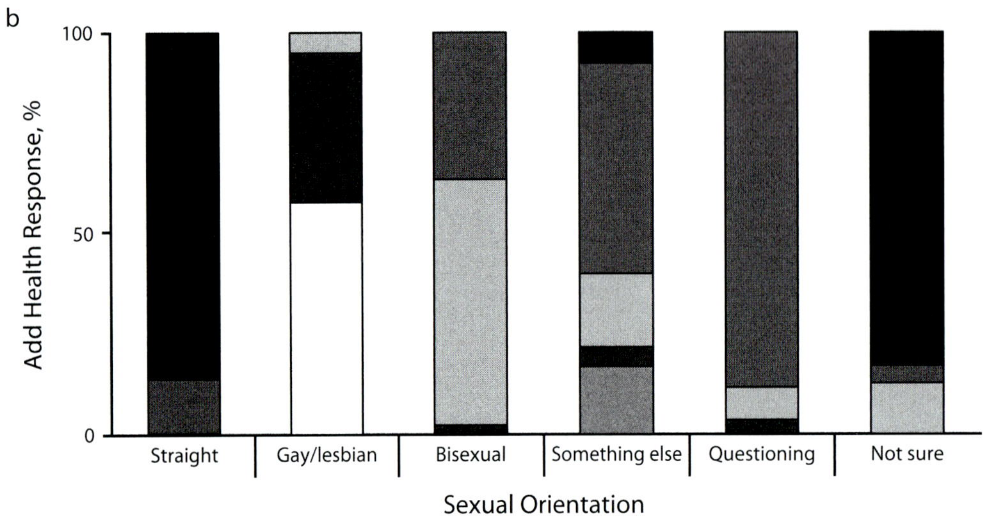

	Straight	Gay/lesbian	Bisexual	Something else	Questioning	Not sure	Total
NHIS response, %	91.2	2.2	4.7	1.0	0.4	0.6	100.0
Add Health response, %							
100% heterosexual	86.1	...	...	7.6	...	83.0	79.1
Mostly heterosexual	13.6	...	36.5	52.4	88.4	4.4	15.0
Bisexual	0.1	5.1	61.2	18.3	8.1	12.7	3.3
Mostly homosexual	...	37.1	2.3	4.9	3.6	...	1.0
100% homosexual	...	57.9	...	...	...	...	1.3
Not attracted to males or females	0.3	...	...	16.8	...	...	0.4

FIGURE 2— Continued

30.2% of heterosexual or straight respondents, 48.4% of sexual minorities, and 51.5% of undetected sexual minorities endorsed a lifetime depression diagnosis. Adjusted Wald tests comparing these proportions indicated that both sexual minorities ($F = 18.49$; $P < .001$) and undetected sexual minorities ($F = 13.91$; $P < .001$) were significantly more likely than heterosexual or straight respondents to endorse a depression diagnosis, and the difference between sexual minorities and undetected sexual minorities was not significantly different ($F = 0.24$; $P = 1.00$). After stratifying by gender, cisgender female sexual minorities (52.2%; $F = 10.42$; $P < .01$) were significantly more likely than cisgender female heterosexual or straight respondents (35.8%) to have ever been

TABLE 1— Sexual Orientation Categories by Question and Gender in the Sexual Orientation/Gender Identity, Socioeconomic Status, and Health Across the Life Course (SOGI-SES) Study: United States, 2020–2021

	Add Health Question			NHIS Question		
	Cisgender Male, %	Cisgender Female, %	Total, %	Cisgender Male, %	Cisgender Female, %	Total, %
Heterosexual or straight	92.2	79.0	85.6	92.2	79.0	85.6
Sexual minority	7.8	20.9	14.4	5.3	8.3	6.8
Undetected sexual minority	< 0.1	< 0.1	< 0.1	2.6	12.8	7.6

Note. Add Health = National Longitudinal Study of Adolescent to Adult Health; NHIS = National Health Interview Study. Percentages are weighted to yield population-representative estimates and may not sum to 100% because of rounding. The sample size was n = 2558.

TABLE 2— Adjusted Wald Tests Comparing Proportions Who Endorsed Ever Receiving Mental Health Diagnoses in the Sexual Orientation/Gender Identity, Socioeconomic Status, and Health Across the Life Course (SOGI-SES) Study, by Sexual Orientation Category and Gender: United States, 2020–2021

	Heterosexual or Straight, % (95% CI)	Sexual Minority, % (95% CI)	Undetected by the NHIS Question, % (95% CI)
Depression			
Cisgender male	25.7 (18.7, 34.1)[a]	42.8 (31.7, 54.6)[b]	47.6 (26.5, 69.6)
Cisgender female	35.8 (29.3, 42.8)[a]	52.2 (43.7, 60.6)[b]	52.3 (41.2, 63.3)
Overall	30.2 (25.0, 36.1)[a,c]	48.4 (41.3, 55.6)[b]	51.5 (41.3, 61.6)[b]
Anxiety or panic disorder			
Cisgender male	30.1 (23.1, 38.1)[a]	46.3 (36.6, 56.3)[b]	42.9 (22.2, 66.5)
Cisgender female	37.1 (30.5, 44.2)[a]	54.7 (46.1, 63.0)[b]	47.6 (37.3, 58.0)
Overall	33.3 (28.2, 38.7)[a]	51.3 (44.8, 57.7)[b]	46.8 (37.3, 56.4)

Note. CI = confidence interval; NHIS=National Health Interview Survey. Gender diverse identity category was excluded because of small cell sizes. Percentages are weighted to yield population representative estimates and may not sum to 100% because of rounding. The sample size was n = 2472.
[a]Statistically significant difference ($P<.05$) from "sexual minority" after the Bonferroni correction.
[b]Statistically significant difference ($P<.05$) from "heterosexual or straight" after the Bonferroni correction.
[c]Statistically significant difference ($P<.05$) from "undetected by the NHIS question" after the Bonferroni correction.

diagnosed with depression. Cisgender females who were undetected sexual minorities (52.3%) were not significantly different from cisgender female heterosexual or straight respondents after the Bonferroni correction for multiple comparisons ($F=5.73$; $P=.05$) or cisgender female sexual minorities ($F=0.00$; $P=1.00$). Among cisgender male respondents, sexual minorities were significantly more likely than heterosexual or straight respondents (42.8% vs 25.7%; $F=6.71$; $P=.03$) to have received a depression diagnosis. No such statistically significant differences in depression diagnosis emerged when comparing cisgender males who were undetected sexual minorities (47.6%) to cisgender male heterosexual or straight respondents ($F=3.63$; $P=.18$) or to cisgender male sexual minorities ($F=0.15$; $P=1.00$).

The overall pattern was similar for anxiety or panic disorder. A total of 33.3% of heterosexual or straight respondents, 51.3% of sexual minorities, and 46.8% of undetected sexual minorities endorsed a lifetime anxiety or panic disorder diagnosis. Adjusted Wald tests showed that sexual minorities were significantly more likely than heterosexual or straight respondents ($F=18.66$; $P<.001$) to have ever been diagnosed with anxiety or panic disorder. Undetected sexual minorities were not significantly different from heterosexual or straight respondents after the Bonferroni correction ($F=5.87$; $P=.05$) or from sexual minorities ($F=0.69$; $P=1.00$). Similarly, after stratifying by gender, the only statistically significant differences in the proportions endorsing an anxiety or panic disorder diagnosis were between sexual minorities and heterosexual or straight respondents among both cisgender male (46.3% vs 30.1%; $F=6.99$; $P=.03$) and cisgender female respondents (54.7% vs 37.1%; $F=10.51$; $P<.01$).

DISCUSSION

As hypothesized, we found that the NHIS survey question detected significantly fewer sexual minority respondents compared with the Add Health survey question. In addition, the mental health outcomes of those who reported being sexual minorities on one question but not the other (e.g., heterosexual or straight to the NHIS question and sexual minority to the Add Health question) were more similar to those who reported being sexual minorities to both questions than to those who reported being heterosexual or straight to both questions. Such findings suggest that a large group of sexual minorities are undetected by measures that offer no options in between heterosexual and bisexual, which may lead to an underestimation of the scope and prevalence of health disparities. Importantly, this research further illustrates the critical need to expand measurement of sexual orientation.[4,19] A singular focus on identity may exclude those who experience same-sex attraction or behaviors who are at similar or greater risk for negative health outcomes, even though they do not identify with a sexual minority label. Therefore, future work in this area should consider (1) testing response options that allow for identification in between straight and bisexual and (2) also measuring current sexual attraction and adult lifetime behavior, in addition to identity, when collecting information about sexuality on health surveys.

Limitations

Study findings should be interpreted within the context of the following limitations. First, sample size limited our ability to detect differences in smaller sexual minority subgroups. Similarly, sample size prevented us from understanding how these patterns may vary by other demographic characteristics such as race and ethnicity. This is particularly important given the large body of research showing significant health inequities experienced by people of color who also identify as lesbian, gay, bisexual, or any other minority sexual orientation.[20,21]

It is also important to acknowledge the limitations of the Add Health sexual orientation question. Importantly, this question asks about both identity and attraction in the same item, which may be interpreted differently and thus lead to less-precise estimates.[3,11] In addition, certain terms, such as "heterosexual" and "homosexual," may be less effective in detecting sexual minority populations as they do not reflect the terms used by more contemporary cohorts.[11] A further limitation is that SOGI-SES respondents have responded to the Add Health question previously, possibly as many as 3 previous times. Present findings may not generalize to samples who are answering a survey question for the first time. Finally, the SOGI-SES study was conducted only in English, so these results do not necessarily represent the experiences of those who are monolingual in other languages. Despite these limitations, the Add Health question did detect a larger sexual minority group that would have otherwise been uncounted, suggesting the importance of including other dimensions of sexual orientation (i.e., attraction, behavior) and approximating a continuum when estimating the size of the sexual minority population.

Public Health Implications

The results of this study show how current 1-dimensional measures of sexual orientation in national-level surveys may lead to underestimates of the sexual minority population and, therefore, further underestimate the significant health disparities they experience. Thus, further research on other measures that consider response options that reflect a broader continuum of sexuality are needed to inform health policy and service planning to meet the needs of the sexual minority population. AJPH

ABOUT THE AUTHORS

Nicole F. Kahn is with the Division of Adolescent Medicine, Department of Pediatrics, School of Medicine, University of Washington, Seattle; Center for Child Health, Behavior and Development, Seattle Children's Research Institute; and Department of Maternal and Child Health, Gillings School of Global Public Health, University of North Carolina at Chapel Hill. Carolyn T. Halpern is with the Department of Maternal and Child Health, Gillings School of Global Public Health; and Carolina Population Center, University of North Carolina at Chapel Hill. Dana R. Burshell is with the Carolina Population Center. Stephanie M. Hernandez is with the Department of Epidemiology and Biostatistics, Dornsife School of Public Health, Drexel University, Philadelphia, PA; Department of Maternal and Child Health, Gillings School of Global Public Health; and Carolina Population Center. Kerith J. Conron is with the Williams Institute, School of Law, University of California Los Angeles, and Carolina Population Center.

CORRESPONDENCE

Correspondence should be sent to Nicole F. Kahn, PhD, MEd, Center for Child Health, Behavior and Development, Seattle Children's Research Institute, 1920 Terry Ave, Seattle, WA 98101 (e-mail: nicole.kahn@seattlechildrens.org). Reprints can be ordered at https://www.ajph.org by clicking the "Reprints" link.

PUBLICATION INFORMATION

Full Citation: Kahn NF, Halpern CT, Burshell DR, Hernandez SM, Conron KJ. Assessment of health disparities and sexual orientation response choices used in two US national population-based health surveys, 2020–2021. *Am J Public Health*. 2024;114(12):1375–1383.

Acceptance Date: August 3, 2024.

DOI: https://doi.org/10.2105/AJPH.2024.307839

ORCID iDs:

Nicole F. Kahn https://orcid.org/0000-0001-6523-7680

Dana R. Burshell https://orcid.org/0000-0001-5519-7590

Stephanie M. Hernandez https://orcid.org/0000-0003-4571-1191

Kerith J. Conron https://orcid.org/0000-0002-1487-2278

CONTRIBUTORS

N. F. Kahn conceptualized and designed the study, analyzed and interpreted the data, and drafted the article. C. T. Halpern conceptualized and designed the study, revised the article for important intellectual content, and provided supervision. D. R. Burshell revised the article for important intellectual content and provided administrative, technical, and logistic support. S. M. Hernandez revised the article for important intellectual content and provided technical and logistic support. K. J. Conron revised the article for important intellectual content and provided supervision. All authors approved the final version of the article for publication.

ACKNOWLEDGMENTS

The Sexual Orientation/Gender Identity, Socioeconomic Status, and Health Across the Life Course (SOGI-SES) Study is co-directed by principal investigators C. T. Halpern at the University of North Carolina at Chapel Hill and K. J. Conron at the Williams Institute, UCLA, and is funded by the Eunice Kennedy Shriver National Institute of Child Health and Human Development (NICHD) and the National Institute on Minority Health and Health Disparities under grants R01 HD087365 and R01 HD087365-03S1. SOGI-SES is an Add Health ancillary study that includes a subset of Add Health respondents. Waves I through V of Add Health were funded by grant P01 HD31921 (Harris) from the NICHD, with cooperative funding from 23 other federal agencies and foundations. Add Health is currently directed by Robert A. Hummer and funded by the National Institute on Aging cooperative agreements U01 AG071448 (Hummer) and U01AG071450 (Aiello and Hummer) at the University of North Carolina at Chapel Hill. Add

Health was designed by J. Richard Udry, Peter S. Bearman, and Kathleen Mullan Harris at the University of North Carolina at Chapel Hill. Research reported in this publication was supported by NICHD of the National Institutes of Health under award P2C HD050924 and the Office of the Director, National Institutes of Health, under grant U54CA267735.

CONFLICTS OF INTEREST

The authors have no conflicts of interest to disclose.

HUMAN PARTICIPANT PROTECTION

This study was reviewed and approved by the institutional review board at the University of North Carolina at Chapel Hill.

REFERENCES

1. Jones J. US LGBT identification steady at 7.2%. 2023. Available at: https://news.gallup.com/poll/470708/lgbt-identification-steady.aspx. Accessed July 11, 2023.
2. Deng B, Watson T. LGBTQ+ data availability: What we can learn from four major surveys. *Policy Commons.* 2023. Available at: https://policycommons.net/artifacts/4137206/lgbtq-data-availability-what-we-can-learn-from-four-major-surveys. Accessed July 11, 2023.
3. National Academies of Sciences, Engineering, and Medicine. *Measuring Sex, Gender Identity, and Sexual Orientation.* Washington, DC: The National Academies Press; 2022.
4. Patterson JG, Jabson JM, Bowen DJ. Measuring sexual and gender minority populations in health surveillance. *LGBT Health.* 2017;4(2):82–105. https://doi.org/10.1089/lgbt.2016.0026
5. National Academies of Sciences, Engineering, and Medicine. *Understanding the Well-Being of LGBTQI+ Populations.* Washington, DC: The National Academies Press; 2020.
6. Meyer IH. Prejudice, social stress, and mental health in lesbian, gay, and bisexual populations: conceptual issues and research evidence. *Psychol Bull.* 2003;129(5):674–697. https://doi.org/10.1037/0033-2909.129.5.674
7. Meyer IH, Frost DM. Minority stress and the health of sexual minorities. In: Patterson CJ, D'Augelli AR, eds. *Handbook of Psychology and Sexual Orientation.* New York, NY: Oxford University Press; 2013:252–266.
8. Frost DM, Meyer IH. Minority stress theory: application, critique, and continued relevance. *Curr Opin Psychol.* 2023;51:101579. https://doi.org/10.1016/j.copsyc.2023.101579
9. Krueger EA, Upchurch DM. Are sociodemographic, lifestyle, and psychosocial characteristics associated with sexual orientation group differences in mental health disparities? Results from a national population-based study. *Soc Psychiatry Psychiatr Epidemiol.* 2019;54(6):755–770. https://doi.org/10.1007/s00127-018-1649-0
10. Vrangalova Z, Savin-Williams RC. Mostly heterosexual and mostly gay/lesbian: evidence for new sexual orientation identities. *Arch Sex Behav.* 2012;41(1):85–101. https://doi.org/10.1007/s10508-012-9921-y
11. Suen LW, Lunn MR, Katuzny K, et al. What sexual and gender minority people want researchers to know about sexual orientation and gender identity questions: a qualitative study. *Arch Sex Behav.* 2020;49(7):2301–2318. https://doi.org/10.1007/s10508-020-01810-y
12. Pachankis JE, Mahon CP, Jackson SD, Fetzner BK, Bränström R. Sexual orientation concealment and mental health: a conceptual and meta-analytic review. *Psychol Bull.* 2020;146(10):831–871. https://doi.org/10.1037/bul0000271
13. Salomaa AC, Matsick JL, Exten C, Kruk M. Different categorizations of women's sexual orientation reveal unique health outcomes in a nationally representative US sample. *Womens Health Issues.* 2023;33(1):87–96. https://doi.org/10.1016/j.whi.2022.07.003
14. Krueger EA, Meyer IH, Upchurch DM. Sexual orientation group differences in perceived stress and depressive symptoms among young adults in the United States. *LGBT Health.* 2018;5(4):242–249. https://doi.org/10.1089/lgbt.2017.0228
15. Harris KM, Halpern CT, Whitsel E, et al. *Add Health Research Design.* Carolina Population Center. 2009. Available at: https://addhealth.cpc.unc.edu/documentation/study-design. Accessed June 21, 2023.
16. Halpern CT, Burshell DR, Hernandez SM, Qu L, Conron KJ. *Sexual Orientation/Gender Identity, Socioeconomic Status, and Health Across the Life Course (SOGI-SES) User Guide.* Carolina Population Center. 2023. Available at: https://addhealth.cpc.unc.edu/sogi-ses-user-guide. Accessed June 21, 2023.
17. Miller K, Ryan JM. *Design, Development, and Testing of the NHIS Sexual Identity Question.* National Center for Health Statistics. 2011. Available at: https://wwwn.cdc.gov/qbank/report/Miller_NCHS_2011_NHIS%20Sexual%20Identity.pdf. Accessed June 21, 2023.
18. Dahlhamer JM, Galinsky AM, Joestl SS, Ward BW. Sexual orientation in the 2013 National Health Interview Survey: a quality assessment. *Vital Health Stat.* 2014;2(169):1–32.
19. Julian CA, Manning WD, Westrick-Payne KK. Responses to sexual and gender identity measures in population-level data by birth cohort: a research note. *Demography.* 2024;61(1):15–30. https://doi.org/10.1215/00703370-11164985
20. Crenshaw K. Mapping the margins: intersectionality, identity politics, and violence against women of color. *Stanford Law Rev.* 1991;43(6):1241–1299. https://doi.org/10.2307/1229039
21. Walubita T, Beccia AL, Boama-Nyarko E, Ding EY, Ferrucci KA, Jesdale BM. Complicating narratives of sexual minority mental health: an intersectional analysis of frequent mental distress at the intersection of sexual orientation, gender identity, and race/ethnicity. *LGBT Health.* 2022;9(3):161–168. https://doi.org/10.1089/lgbt.2021.0099

Levels and Changes in Defensive Firearm Use by US Crime Victims, 1987–2021

David McDowall, PhD, Brian Wiersema, BA, Colin Loftin, PhD, and Richard McCleary, PhD

AJPH December 2024, Vol. 114, No. 12

Objectives. To examine levels and temporal changes in the frequency of defensive gun use by US crime victims.

Methods. We computed national-level counts of criminal incidents involving firearm defense during 3 periods: 1993 to 2005, 2007 to 2015, and 2016 to 2021. We also considered earlier national estimates for 1987 to 1990. The data came from the US Bureau of Justice Statistics National Crime Victimization Survey (NCVS). We counted firearm defenses as incidents in which victims used a gun to threaten or attack an offender.

Results. Over the 4 periods, for all crimes, victims reported gun defenses in an average range of between 61 000 and 65 000 incidents per year. This included between 38 000 and 53 000 personal (violent) incidents and between 12 000 and 23 000 household (property) incidents.

Conclusions. Firearm defenses occurred at a relatively low and nearly constant level over the 35-year period. Although some victims use guns for defense, these uses are infrequent compared with the incidence of crime.

Public Health Implications. The continuing relative rarity of NCVS armed defenses suggests that claims about the protective benefits of widespread firearm ownership may be overstated. (*Am J Public Health*. 2024;114(12):1384–1387. https://doi.org/10.2105/AJPH.2024.307838)

How often crime victims use guns for self-defense is an issue in firearm policy research. General gun ownership carries well-documented social costs, including deaths and injuries from criminal misuse.[1,2] Yet armed victims may avoid personal harms, and guns may help deter would-be offenders.[2,3] Opponents of measures that might affect firearm access stress these possibilities and argue that armed defenses occur as often as several million times each year.[3,4]

Multiple estimates of the frequency of defensive gun use exist, but most of these are 20 to 30 years old.[2,3] The estimates also come from cross-sectional analyses, and methodological differences limit comparisons between them. Few studies present recent data, and none, to our knowledge, examine changes in firearm defenses over time.

We used the National Crime Victimization Survey (NCVS) to examine the frequency of defensive gun use. The NCVS provides annual estimates of the incidence of crime in the United States, and its core methodology has remained constant over time.[5,6] Our goal was to update earlier NCVS estimates of firearm defense and to assess temporal variations.

METHODS

The NCVS uses a multistage probability sample of US housing units. The US Census Bureau conducts the survey for the US Bureau of Justice Statistics (BJS). In 2021, the sample consisted of about 150 000 housing units, occupied by 240 000 persons. Housing units remain in the NCVS for 3.5 years, and, at 6-month intervals, residents aged 12 years or older answer screening questions about their experiences with crime. Respondents who report attempted or completed victimizations provide additional details. The NCVS collects information on personal crimes (rape, robbery, assault, and personal larceny) and household crimes (burglary and trespassing, household larceny, and motor vehicle theft).[6]

If victims say that they saw an offender, NCVS interviewers ask, "Did you do anything with the idea of protecting yourself or your property while the incident was going on?" If respondents report no protective actions, interviewers rephrase the question and ask it again. Respondents who offer positive responses next describe what they did. The interviewers code the descriptions into categories that include "attacked offender with gun; fired gun" and "threatened offender with gun."[5]

Our estimates are incident counts, weighted to represent the population at risk.[6] The estimates for personal crimes represent the resident noninstitutional population of the United States, aged 12 years or older. The estimates for household crimes represent US housing units. We computed standard errors for the estimates using the BJS's generalized variance formulas.[6]

As we show in the Results section, firearm defenses are rare, making annual estimates highly variable. To increase stability, we aggregated incidents into 3 periods: 1993 to 2005, 2007 to 2015, and 2016 to 2021. We selected these aggregations partly because they contain many sample cases and partly because they align with changes in the survey. Budget-related modifications in data collection and sample revisions following the 2000 Census produced anomalous 2006 estimates.[6] The BJS recommends against using the 2006 data, and breaking the series after 2005 allows its exclusion. Another series break occurred in 2016, with changes to sample sites and interview staff based on the 2010 Census.[6]

Besides 1993 to 2021, we also included previously published estimates covering 1987 to 1990.[7] These use an earlier version of the survey, before the BJS revised the screening questions to encourage more reports. The sample designs and question structures are almost identical across the versions, however, and with cautious interpretations, the earlier estimates supply useful information.

RESULTS

Period-specific estimates of defensive gun use appear in Table 1. Since most defenses involve personal crimes, the table presents both total estimates and separate estimates for personal and household offenses. Assuming an even annual distribution of incidents within aggregations, total defenses ranged between about 61 000 and 65 000 per year, giving an impression of near-constancy over the 35-year period.

Similar results appear after separating personal and household crimes. These estimates are more variable, but in all periods, armed defenses occurred with roughly similar frequencies. Victimizations have decreased in the NCVS overall, slightly raising the proportion of defensive incidents. The proportions are nevertheless uniformly small, exceeding 1% of personal incidents in 2016 to 2021 and falling below 1% for the other aggregations.

DISCUSSION

Between 1987 and 2021, the NCVS yields a stable estimate of about 61 000 to 65 000 defensive gun incidents per year. One should not dismiss firearms as a defense against crime, but armed defenses are infrequent compared with the total volume of offenses or the subset of offenses involving guns. In the 3 periods between 1993 and 2021, the NCVS produces an estimate of 13 062 630 nonfatal firearm crimes. This is 7.3 times larger than our estimate of 1 792 308 armed defenses during the same interval.

Over the analysis period, many states have relaxed laws against carrying guns or have enacted "stand your ground" laws to support resistance against criminal attacks.[8,9] Also during this period, however, opportunities for armed defenses have decreased. Personal victimizations fell from 79.8 per 1000 (in 1993) to 16.5 per 1000 (in 2021), and household victimizations decreased from 322 to 90.3 per 1000.[6] These lower rates may offset any effects of policies that encourage gun use.

The NCVS is not the only source of information about armed defense, and private surveys provide estimates of its frequency that range from 600 000 to 6.1 million incidents annually.[3] The source of the divergence from the NCVS is a longstanding issue, and extensive discussions of the matter exist in the research literature.[1,2] The Appendix (available as a supplement to the online version of this article at https://ajph.org) summarizes the debate.

Although opinions vary, one explanation of the difference lies in the questions that the surveys pose. The NCVS asks about defense only after respondents have reported an attempted or completed crime. Although the other surveys differ in their exact question wordings, all ask a variation on the following: "Have you yourself or another member of your household used a gun, even if it was not fired, for self-protection or for the protection of property at home, work, or elsewhere?"

TABLE 1— Estimates of Number of Self-Defensive Firearm Incidents, All Crimes, Personal Crimes, and Household Crimes, Using National Crime Victimization Survey Data: United States, 1987–2021

Period	Total Firearm Defense Incidents for Period, No. (SE)	Mean Firearm Defense Incidents per Year	Percentage of All Criminal Incidents With Firearm Defense
All crimes			
1987–1990	258 460 (41 012)	64 615	0.18
1993–2005	850 617 (85 674)	65 432	0.21
2007–2015	550 379 (62 558)	61 153	0.30
2016–2021	391 312 (56 432)	65 219	0.39
Personal crimes only			
1987–1990	192 539 (32 394)	48 135	0.83
1993–2005	692 310 (33 255)	53 255	0.73
2007–2015	340 968 (35 552)	37 885	0.81
2016–2021	262 213 (30 438)	43 702	1.04
Household crimes only			
1987–1990	65 921 (18 107)	16 480	0.05
1993–2005	158 307 (17 810)	12 177	0.05
2007–2015	209 311 (35 849)	23 257	0.13
2016–2021	129 099 (21 929)	21 516	0.17

Source. 1987–1990 estimates were adapted from Table 1 from McDowall and Wiersema[7] and use a different version of the survey than do the others.

This question asks about gun use without first establishing the existence of a criminal act, and it relies on respondents' perceptions of intent. It allows respondents to include gun uses to forestall perceived imminent victimizations, and these may sometimes amount to crimes themselves.

A National Academy of Sciences report on the matter characterized the NCVS and non-NCVS questions as different definitions of defense: "as a response to victimization or as a means to prevent victimization from occurring in the first place."[2(p102)] In line with this difference, survey experiments find that the non-NCVS questions generate many more gun use reports than does the NCVS approach.[10,11] A limitation of the NCVS is that it does not directly ask respondents about gun use, instead recording it when they describe it as a response to victimization. This feature aside, we believe that the NCVS better aligns with common understandings of self-defense.

PUBLIC HEALTH IMPLICATIONS

Self-defense against crime is the major stated reason for US gun ownership.[12] Crime victims do use firearms for defense, and, as measured by the NCVS, the frequency of defense has been steady over the last 35 years. Yet, also according to the NCVS, gun defenses are rare compared against the volume of crime. This suggests caution in accepting claims of millions of firearm defenses per year. AJPH

ABOUT THE AUTHORS

David McDowall and Colin Loftin are with the School of Criminal Justice and the Violence Research Group, University at Albany–State University of New York (SUNY), Albany, NY. Brian Wiersema is with the Violence Research Group, University at Albany–SUNY. Richard McCleary is with the Department of Criminology, Law, and Society, School of Social Ecology, University of California, Irvine.

CORRESPONDENCE

Correspondence should be sent to David McDowall, School of Criminal Justice, University at Albany–SUNY, 135 Western Ave, Albany, NY 12222 (e-mail: dmcdowall@albany.edu). Reprints can be ordered at https://www.ajph.org by clicking the "Reprints" link.

PUBLICATION INFORMATION

Full Citation: McDowall D, Wiersema B, Loftin C, McCleary R. Levels and changes in defensive firearm use by US crime victims, 1987–2021. *Am J Public Health*. 2024;114(12):1384–1387.
Acceptance Date: August 3, 2024.
DOI: https://doi.org/10.2105/AJPH.2024.307838

CONTRIBUTORS

D. McDowall conceptualized the study, interpreted the results, and wrote the article. B. Wiersema curated the data and conducted the analyses. C. Loftin and R. McCleary conceptualized the study. All authors critically reviewed and commented on the article.

CONFLICTS OF INTEREST

The authors have no conflicts of interest to report.

HUMAN PARTICIPANT PROTECTION

All data in this study are available in the public domain and did not require institutional review board approval.

REFERENCES

1. Hemenway D. *Private Guns, Public Health*. New ed. Ann Arbor, MI: University of Michigan Press; 2017.
2. National Research Council; Wellford CF, Pepper JV, Petrie CV, eds. *Firearms and Violence: A Critical Review*. Washington, DC: National Academies Press; 2005.
3. Kleck G. What do CDC's surveys say about the prevalence of defensive gun use? *Am J Crim Justice*. 2020;46(3):401–421. https://doi.org/10.1007/s12103-020-09562-0
4. LaPierre W. CDC: the centers for disinformation and censorship. *America's 1st Freedom*. February 21, 2023. Available at: https://www.americas1stfreedom.org/content/standing-guard-cdc-the-centers-for-disinformation-and-censorship. Accessed September 11, 2024.
5. US Bureau of Justice Statistics. National Crime Victimization Survey, Concatenated File, [United States], 1992–2021. Ann Arbor, MI: Inter-university Consortium for Political and Social Research; September 19, 2022. https://doi.org/10.3886/ICPSR38430.v1
6. *Criminal Victimization, 2021*. Washington, DC: US Bureau of Justice Statistics; 2022.
7. McDowall D, Wiersema B. The incidence of defensive firearm use by US crime victims, 1987 through 1990. *Am J Public Health*. 1994;84(12):1982–1984. https://doi.org/10.2105/AJPH.84.12.1982
8. Siegel M, Xuan Z, Ross CS, et al. Easiness of legal access to concealed firearm permits and homicide rates in the United States. *Am J Public Health*. 2017;107(12):1923–1929. https://doi.org/10.2105/AJPH.2017.304057
9. Degli Esposti M, Wiebe DJ, Gasparrini A, Humphreys DK. Analysis of "stand your ground" self-defense laws and statewide rates of homicides and firearm homicides. *JAMA Netw Open*. 2022;5(2):e220077. https://doi.org/10.1001/jamanetworkopen.2022.0077
10. McDowall D, Loftin C, Presser S. Measuring civilian defensive firearm use: a methodological experiment. *J Quant Criminol*. 2000;16(1):1–19. https://doi.org/10.1023/A:1007588410221
11. Kleck G. Response errors in survey estimates of defensive gun use: a national Internet survey experiment. *Crime Delinq*. 2018;64(9):1119–1142. https://doi.org/10.1177/0011128718763138
12. For most US gun owners, protection is the main reason they own a gun. Washington, DC: Pew Research Center; August 2023.

Employer Demand and Desired Skills for Public Health Graduates: Evidence From Job Postings

Heather Krasna, PhD, EdM, MS

See also Magaña and Burke, p. 1298.

Objectives. To determine whether job postings from employers seeking master of public health (MPH) graduates require skills aligning with Council on Education in Public Health (CEPH) competencies.

Methods. I analyzed a data set of 70 343 job postings in the United States for MPH graduates from Lightcast, a data vendor that collects, cleans, and analyzes millions of job postings per year. I contrasted skills from the postings with CEPH competencies.

Results. Most postings were from for-profit industry, academia and research, or hospitals and health care, with only 12% from government. The skills from job postings aligned well with CEPH competencies, but some CEPH competencies did not appear in the top skills in job postings.

Conclusions. Although accredited public health degree programs provide key competencies demanded by employers, they can improve graduate employability by ensuring that their graduates also obtain specific technical skills listed in job postings. (*Am J Public Health*. 2024;114(12):1388–1393. https://doi.org/10.2105/AJPH.2024.307834)

AJPH December 2024, Vol. 114, No. 12

The master of public health (MPH) is a professional degree designed to prepare graduates to succeed in a specific field. Although accredited schools and programs of public health are required to gather input from employers as part of the accreditation process, the actual competencies required for the MPH curriculum are established by the Council on Education in Public Health (CEPH).[1] These competencies are drawn from several sources, including the Council on Linkages Between Academia and Public Health Practice Core Competencies for Public Health Professionals, "a consensus set of knowledge and skills for the broad practice of public health, as defined by the 10 Essential Public Health Services."[2] The most recent of these lists of competencies, formulated in 2021, was created through a review process that involved town hall meetings and discussions and requests for comments. Other competency frameworks in public health are the de Beaumont Foundation's Strategic Skills[3] and the National Board of Public Health Examiners' Job Task Analysis, which is used to collect skills for the Certified in Public Health Examination.[4]

Sets of cross-cutting skills or competencies for public health professionals tend to draw primarily from the governmental public health workforce, but only approximately 19% of MPH graduates find employment in this sector.[5] Further complicating the issue of designing MPH programs for cross-cutting competencies is that there are approximately 73 distinct occupations in the governmental public health workforce—each of which may require different competencies—but only about 17% of this workforce has an MPH degree.[6,7]

If most competency information comes from a sector that employs only 19% of MPH graduates but also hires many different types of workers who do not require an MPH degree, how accurate are the CEPH competencies in terms of assessing what the majority of current employers require from MPH graduates?

One way to gather direct information about competencies, knowledge, skills, and abilities that employers require is to analyze job descriptions, a method used in several other studies in public health.[8–13] Job descriptions must be approved by the human resources department of an employer organization and should include detailed information on the essential functions for the role to adhere to employment laws. I sought to determine whether the current CEPH competencies align with job requirements listed in recent job postings from employers seeking to hire MPH graduates.

METHODS

Drawing on past research using job descriptions to assess required skills and employer types for public health graduates, I conducted a study using data from Lightcast, a large-scale data vendor that gathers job postings from tens of thousands of sites and aggregates, deduplicates, and analyzes "between 6 and 8 million unique, active postings from more than 90 000 companies"[14] each month.[8,11] I conducted a search of Lightcast on July 16, 2023 for jobs posted in the United States between July 2022 and February 2023 requiring or preferring a master's degree in the Classification of Instructional Program's Codes for Public Health (51.22) and all of its subcodes, such as Public Health Education and Promotion (51.2207), International Public Health/International Health (51.2210), Health Services Administration (51.2211), Maternal and Child Health (51.2209), Environmental Health (51.2202), Occupational Health and Industrial Hygiene (51.2206), Community Health and Preventive Medicine (51.2208), Behavioral Aspects of Health (51.2212), and Epidemiology (26.1309). I excluded jobs requiring a registered nurse credential. I excluded the Biostatistics Classification of Instructional Program code for this study because of a large number of job postings that were less relevant to public health.

Lightcast uses machine learning and natural language processing tools to deduplicate job postings; code the job postings by occupation type, job title, company name, industry, and skills; and provide a list of salary ranges. Lightcast assesses job postings for word sequences that suggest skills and matches them to a "comprehensive taxonomy of over 32 000 . . . skills collected from hundreds of millions of job postings, resumes, and online profiles"[14] to categorize skills. Skills are organized into common skills, which are common among many occupations and include soft skills and competencies (e.g., communication or problem-solving); specialized skills, which are technical or hard skills that qualify candidates for certain subsets of occupations (e.g., Java or financial analysis competency); software skills; and certifications and licenses (e.g., radiological nurse certification). Lightcast also uses a list of more than 75 000 job titles. Job titles refer to the specific name given to a particular job role, and an occupation is a broader term referring to what individuals in a group of related roles, potentially with multiple job titles, actually do in terms of job tasks. Skills are used to describe job tasks and competencies required for particular occupations.

Although "skills" and "competencies" are often used interchangeably, the Council on Linkages describes its core competencies as a "set of knowledge and skills." Competencies can be construed as a grouping of attributes combining multiple abilities, knowledge, behaviors, attitudes, and skills; whereas skills describe a single proficiency. For example, the competency in data analytics and assessment includes multiple skills, such as identifying data, collecting data, and understanding data.

I used a thematic approach to qualitatively match CEPH competencies and competency categories with the skills from the job postings; for example, I identified word matches between the words for Lightcast skills and wording in the CEPH competency statements. I then contrasted the top Lightcast skills requirements for these job postings with the CEPH competencies to find areas of alignment or gaps. I also reviewed the Lightcast results to assess which employers, industries, occupations, and job titles were most common.

RESULTS

There were approximately 70 343 unique job postings in the report (the numbers of job postings listed varied in each of the subreports because of how Lightcast categorized the data). Of these, 33 620 listed a salary range; the median advertised salary was $76 672. The job postings required a range of experience, with 20.6% not listing any experience requirement, 8.5% requiring zero to 1 year of experience, 26.1% requiring 2 to 3 years of experience, 29.4% requiring 4 to 6 years of experience, 8.6% requiring 7 to 9 years, and 6.9% requiring 10 or more years.

The most common job titles listed are shown in full in Table A (available as a supplement to the online version of this article at http://www.ajph.org). These were epidemiologists, biostatisticians, environmental health and safety specialists, program managers, nurse epidemiologists, data analysts, industrial hygienists, principal biostatisticians, project managers, data scientists, medical directors, IT (information technology) analysts, and environmental health and safety managers.

The top 20 employer companies were health insurance and managed care firms (e.g., Elevance Health, Humana, UnitedHealth Group, and Centene), universities (e.g., University of California, Johns Hopkins University, Indiana University, University of Michigan, University of Colorado), consulting firms (e.g., Guidehouse and Evolent Health), contract research organizations (e.g., Parexel and Mathematica Policy Research), technology firms (e.g., Amazon), external quality review organizations (e.g., Health Services Advisory Group), health care companies and hospitals (e.g., Kaiser Permanente, Highmark Health, and Emory Healthcare), pharmaceutical firms (e.g., Pfizer), and government agencies (e.g., the State of Louisiana; Table B, available as a supplement to the online version of this article at http://www.ajph.org).

The largest industries (categorized by North American Industry Classification System codes) by total number of unique job postings are listed in Table C (available as a supplement to the online version of this article at http://www.ajph.org): academic institutions (24.1% of all unique postings), insurance companies (9.6%), general medical and surgical hospitals (7.8%), other general government support (a broad category for government agencies; 6.7%), administrative management and general management consulting services (4.9%), and pharmaceutical preparation manufacturing (4.8%).

I analyzed job postings to assess the top specialized skills, common skills, computer and software skills, and certifications. There were 150 skills or certifications across all domains. Most skills were listed as individual words or short phrases, such as "communication" and "data analysis," whereas CEPH competencies included several sentences describing each competency and giving examples of how the competency should be addressed in public health curricula. I qualitatively matched these skills with CEPH competencies and domains by searching for words or phrases in common between the skills and the CEPH competencies, looking up definitions of the skills words or phrases to find overlap with CEPH competency descriptions, or both.

CEPH lists 22 competencies in 8 domains: evidence-based approaches to public health, public health and health care systems, planning and management to promote health, policy in public health, leadership, communication, interprofessional or intersectoral practice, and systems thinking (Table 1; Table D, available as a supplement to the online version of this article at http://www.ajph.org).

Most CEPH competencies or competency categories clearly matched required skills from job descriptions. For example, the Lightcast skills of analysis, epidemiology, and statistical analysis matched CEPH competency number 1: "1. Apply epidemiological methods to settings and situations in public health practice." Lightcast skills (e.g., economics, policy, and social studies; law, regulation, and compliance; and policy analysis, research, and development) matched the policy in public health CEPH competency category.

The competencies with the largest number of job posting to Lightcast skill matches were "19. Communicate audience-appropriate (i.e., nonacademic, nonpeer audience) public health content, both in writing and through oral presentation," which matched 11 job posting skills and "3. Analyze quantitative and qualitative data using biostatistics, informatics, computer-based programming and software, as appropriate," matching 9 skills; as well as "2. Select quantitative and qualitative data collection methods appropriate for a given public health context"; "16. Apply leadership and/or management principles to address a relevant issue"; and "5. Compare the organization, structure and function of health care, public health, and regulatory systems across national and international settings," each matching 4 job posting skills.

However, several CEPH competencies did not clearly match skills from the job descriptions:

> 4. Interpret results of data analysis for public health research, policy or practice [although this could match skills such as analysis]. . . .
> 6. Discuss the means by which structural bias, social inequities and racism undermine health and create challenges to achieving health equity at organizational, community, and systemic levels. . . .
> 13. Propose strategies to identify stakeholders and build coalitions and partnerships for influencing public health outcomes. . . .
> 14. Advocate for political, social or economic policies and programs that will improve health in diverse populations. . . .
> 17. Apply negotiation and mediation skills to address organizational or community challenges. . . .
> 18. Select communication strategies for different audiences and sectors. . . . [and]
> 21. Integrate perspectives from other sectors and/or professions to promote and advance population health.[1]

With a search of the skills taxonomy in Lightcast, I found there are specific skills in the Lightcast skills list that could have matched the CEPH competencies but did not appear in the job postings. These were specialized skills (i.e., diversity and inclusion, health equity, health advocacy, stakeholder engagement, health policy analysis) and common skills (i.e., negotiation, diversity awareness, advocacy, and collaboration).

Conversely, a large number of specific certifications (e.g., certified health

TABLE 1— Top Job Posting Skills From Lightcast Job Postings for MPH Graduates, With Number of Job Postings: United States, 2022–2023

Example Qualification or Skill by Lightcast Category	Total Postings with Qualification, No.
Common skills	
Communications	57 662
Management	50 145
Research	46 248
Leadership	43 431
Writing	34 300
Qualification	
Valid driver's license	11 508
MBA	9 639
Board certified/board eligible	2 417
Certified safety professional	2 258
CPR certification	2 218
Skill subcategories	
Initiative and leadership	77 209
Communication	75 060
General science and research	58 520
Critical thinking and problem-solving	58 252
Public health and disease prevention	56 612
Software skills	
Microsoft Excel	20 663
Microsoft PowerPoint	15 716
Microsoft Office	14 553
SAS (statistical software)	14 428
R (programming language)	10 937
Top skill categories	
Physical and inherent abilities	90 980
Health care	88 924
Business	86 331
Media and communications	84 329
Science and research	71 419

Note. CPR = cardiopulmonary resuscitation; MBA = master of business administration; MPH = master of public health.

education specialist, certified industrial hygienist, certified safety professional, project management professional certification), vague common skills (e.g., detail oriented, customer service, general science and research), and specific computer skills (with, e.g., MS Excel, PowerPoint, SAS, R, Python) did not directly match CEPH competencies.

DISCUSSION

Overall, CEPH competencies appeared to match skills from job postings for public health graduates. It is noteworthy that job postings from employers seeking to hire MPH graduates did not appear to prioritize diversity and inclusion, health equity, policy, advocacy, and other related skills that are CEPH required competencies. There are several possible explanations for this. It is possible that the large proportion of job postings in for-profit corporations (26.3%), health care and hospitals (14.1%), and academia or research (26.4%) and the relative scarcity of job postings in government or nonprofits (~12%) as well as the skewing of job titles toward analytical, technical, and epidemiological roles meant that technical and statistical skills were more in demand than skills in community partnerships and diversity.

Alternatively, although Lightcast's machine-learning algorithms are proprietary, it is possible that its scanning of postings for skills excludes statements in job postings regarding diversity and inclusion, which often appear in sections of the job posting that are separate from the job requirements or duties listed. Even if health equity skills are not listed as the top requirements in job postings, graduates with training in health equity will bring these skills to employers seeking a public health perspective in their workplace. Because health equity is at the center of the essential public health services, ensuring public health graduates receive these skills is crucial, regardless of where graduates find jobs.

Regarding the highly specific computer skills and certifications desired by employers who hire people with an MPH, it is not surprising that these are not listed by name as CEPH competencies. Competencies are constructed as broader reaching than skills. Certain computer skills are generally included or expected as prerequisites in various courses in an MPH program, and these technical skill requirements may rapidly change as technology changes, so it seems appropriate that CEPH does not list them as competencies.

Although CEPH aims to maintain broad-based competencies that can withstand the test of time, public health schools and programs could benefit from ensuring that their graduates gain the specific, current technical skills listed in this study when preparing their students for employment after graduation.

A total of 12% of unique job postings were in government agencies, illustrating ongoing labor market competition for public health graduates from other sectors, especially from higher-paying industries, such as consulting, insurance, and pharmaceuticals.[15] The job market for MPH graduates seems to continue moving toward for-profit companies, such as insurance firms, as well as health care and research or academia, a finding that seems to align with other research findings on employment outcomes of public health graduates.[5,16] It may be useful for schools and programs of public health to consider which employer organizations are hiring the largest number of graduates with the degrees they are offering when helping graduates find employment. Additionally, although CEPH competencies appear to be well aligned with current employer demands, it could benefit the design of future CEPH competencies to ensure that feedback is obtained from industries that hire the largest numbers of graduates.

Limitations

Lightcast uses proprietary tools to code jobs and gather skills information, making interpretations and validations of its analysis challenging. Job postings are not meant for research. Competencies are meant to be broader and more cross-cutting than specific skills or certifications. The job postings included jobs for which an MPH is either required or preferred. It is possible that many if not most of the job postings would be open to candidates with other qualifications or degrees in other disciplines.

Conclusions

Accredited schools and programs of public health generally seem to meet the needs of employers seeking to hire their graduates but can use real-time data from employer job postings to ensure that their graduates meet current employer needs, especially with regard to specific technical skills. CEPH can also expand the sources used to gather data to create lists of competencies by ensuring that feedback is gathered from a diverse range of employers currently hiring public health graduates.

Implications for Policy and Practice

Employers currently seeking to hire MPH graduates are predominantly in for-profit industry, academia and research, and health care. Public health schools and programs can ensure that their graduates are prepared for this current workforce by using data from current job postings. CEPH competencies are generally in alignment with current employer needs. AJPH

ABOUT THE AUTHOR

Heather Krasna is with the Mailman School of Public Health, Columbia University, New York, NY.

CORRESPONDENCE

Correspondence should be sent to Heather Krasna, 722 W. 168 St, New York, NY 10032 (e-mail: hk2778@cumc.columbia.edu). Reprints can be ordered at https://www.ajph.org by clicking the “Reprints” link.

PUBLICATION INFORMATION

Full Citation: Krasna H. Employer demand and desired skills for public health graduates: evidence from job postings. *Am J Public Health*. 2024;114(12):1388–1393.

Acceptance Date: July 30, 2024.

DOI: https://doi.org/10.2105/AJPH.2024.307834

ORCID iD:

Heather Krasna https://orcid.org/0000-0002-4820-9773

ACKNOWLEDGMENTS

I thank J. P. Leider at University of Minnesota for assistance with accessing Lightcast data.

CONFLICTS OF INTEREST

The author has no conflicts of interest to declare.

HUMAN PARTICIPANT PROTECTION

This study was exempt from review because data were job postings and no human participants were involved.

REFERENCES

1. Council on Education for Public Health. About. Available at: https://ceph.org/about/org-info. Accessed March 28, 2021.
2. Public Health Foundation. Core competencies for public health professionals. Available at: http://www.phf.org/resourcestools/pages/core_public_health_competencies.aspx. Accessed January 18, 2021.
3. de Beaumont Foundation. Strategic skills. Available at: https://debeaumont.org/strategic-skills. Accessed August 21, 2022.
4. Kurz RS, Yager C, Yager JD, Foster A, Breidenbach DH, Irwin Z. Advancing the certified in public health examination: a job task analysis. *Public Health Rep*. 2017;132(4):518–523. https://doi.org/10.1177/0033354917710015
5. Plepys CM, Krasna H, Leider JP, Burke EM, Blakely CH, Magaña L. First-destination outcomes for 2015–2018 public health graduates: focus on employment. *Am J Public Health*. 2021;111(3):475–484. https://doi.org/10.2105/AJPH.2020.306038
6. Krasna H, Venkataraman M, Robins M, Patino I, Leider J. Standard occupational classification codes: gaps in federal data on the public health workforce. *Am J Public Health*. 2024;114(1):48–56. https://doi.org/10.2105/AJPH.2023.307463.
7. Leider JP, Harper E, Bharthapudi K, Castrucci BC. Educational attainment of the public health workforce and its implications for workforce development. *J Public Health Manag Pract*. 2015;21(suppl 6):S56–S68. https://doi.org/10.1097/PHH.0000000000000306
8. Krasna H, Czabanowska K, Jiang S, et al. The future of careers at the intersection of climate change and public health: what can job postings and an employer survey tell us? *Int J Environ Res Public Health*. 2020;17(4):1310. https://doi.org/10.3390/ijerph17041310
9. Krasna H, Kulik PKG, Karnik H, Leider JP. Recruiting new talent for public health jobs with evidence-based job descriptions and attractive job postings. *J Public Health Manag Pract*. 2023;29(5):E162–E168. https://doi.org/10.1097/PHH.0000000000001776

10. Watts RD, Bowles DC, Fisher C, Li IW. Public health job advertisements in Australia and New Zealand: a changing landscape. *Aust N Z J Public Health.* 2019;43(6):522–528. https://doi.org/10.1111/1753-6405.12931

11. Krasna H, Czabanowska K, Beck A, Cushman LF, Leider JP. Labour market competition for public health graduates in the United States: a comparison of workforce taxonomies with job postings before and during the COVID-19 pandemic. *Int J Health Plann Manage.* 2021;36(suppl 1):151–167. https://doi.org/10.1002/hpm.3128

12. Frankenfeld CL. Trends in employer postings for epidemiology jobs: an analysis of publichealthjobs.net data from 2003 to 2016. *Ann Epidemiol.* 2017;27(9):553–557.e1. https://doi.org/10.1016/j.annepidem.2017.08.007

13. Cherniak W, Nezami E, Eichbaum Q, et al. Employment opportunities and experiences among recent master's-level global health graduates. *Ann Glob Health.* 2019;85(1):31. https://doi.org/10.5334/aogh.305

14. Lightcast. Lightcast data. Available at: https://lightcast.io/about/data. Accessed July 10, 2023.

15. Krasna H, Leider J, Martin S, Orr J, Venkataraman M, Patino I. Salary disparities in public health occupations: evidence from job postings and salary surveys. 2023. Available at: https://apha.confex.com/apha/2023/meetingapp.cgi/Paper/532508. Accessed December 21, 2023.

16. Krasna H, Kornfeld J, Cushman L, Ni S, Antoniou P, March D. The new public health workforce: employment outcomes of public health graduate students. *J Public Health Manag Pract.* 2021;27(1):12–19. https://doi.org/10.1097/PHH.0000000000000097

More Than 1.4 Million US Children Have Lost a Family Member to Drug Overdose

Ashton M. Verdery, PhD, MA, Cayley Ryan-Claytor, MA, Emily Smith-Greenaway, PhD, MA, Nilakshi Sarkar, BA, and Michelle Livings, PhD, MPH

Objectives. To estimate children's exposure to family overdose in the United States.

Methods. We used recent demographic kinship modeling advances and the Centers for Disease Control and Prevention's most recent underlying cause of death estimates to model how many children aged younger than 18 years in 2019 had lost 1 or more parents, siblings, grandparents, aunts or uncles, or cousins to overdose mortality since birth. We calculated the number and proportion of children with such exposures and considered age, cohort, and gender patterning.

Results. More than 1.4 million children in the United States, mostly adolescents, experienced a family overdose death, often losing central figures like parents or grandparents. Cohort analyses suggest dramatic increases in these exposures, portending mounting prevalence.

Conclusions. Attention to the large population with lives disrupted by overdose deaths should include affected children. The long-arm consequences of the overdose crisis will continue to define the public health landscape for decades. (*Am J Public Health*. 2024;114(12):1394–1397. https://doi.org/10.2105/AJPH.2024.307847)

AJPH December 2024, Vol. 114, No. 12

A recent *AJPH* study by Athey et al. shows that personal connections to overdose deaths have disrupted the lives of more than 1 in 8 adults in the United States.[1] Using survey reports, their study builds on emerging research about the secondary impacts of overdose deaths. Other surveys indicate that 13% of adults lost a loved one or close friend[2] and 9% lost someone in their family[3] to overdose. Collectively, these studies draw attention to a neglected and vulnerable population bereaved by overdose, but they overlook an important group: children younger than 18 years old.

The prevalence of personal connections to overdose loss among children is unclear. Few surveys measure child bereavement in general, let alone children's exposure to specific causes such as overdose. Yet there are many reasons to suspect that exposure to overdose deaths is pervasive among children. The average age of overdose death has drifted down in recent decades,[4] putting those dying of overdose in prime family years. Postpartum overdoses are soaring,[5] amid an exponential expansion in overdose deaths at all ages, including a 12-fold increase since 2000 among adults older than 55 years, that potentially implicates grandparental and other losses.[6] During the same period, long-standing negative associations between family structure and substance use attenuated, also increasing children's risk of loss.[7] Recent modeling efforts confirm these suspicions, finding that 322 000 US children lost a coresidential parent to overdose between 2011 and 2021[8] and 759 000 lost a parent to overdose between 1999 and 2020.[9] Both estimates, however, are cumulated over many years and pertain to the exposure of children who were younger than 18 years at the time of loss, not all of whom remain so. Other familial exposures to overdose loss have not been examined.

Overdose loss among children is severely disruptive. Experiencing a loved one's death profoundly influences immediate and long-term mental and physical health.[10] Children are not immune to these losses; they exhibit a range of behavioral and health challenges after experiencing a family member's death,[11] including elevated rates of substance use.[12] Although most child bereavement research focuses on parental death, other family deaths are also consequential, including siblings[13] and more extended relatives like grandparents, aunts and uncles, and cousins.[14] Children who lose loved ones to stigmatized causes such as overdose face unique risks.[15] Given the critical implications of overdose death for children's short- and long-term well-being, research is needed to establish the prevalence of overdose loss during this key developmental stage.

METHODS

To examine US children's exposure to familial overdose deaths, we modeled whether US children had a relative die from drug or alcohol overdose as an underlying cause of death since birth (see Appendix, available as a supplement to the online version of this article at http://www.ajph.org). Using demographic models of kinship and bereavement and dynamic fertility and mortality data from 2000 to 2019, the most recently available years without COVID-19 disruption, we estimated children's age-by-year exposure to overdose losses among a wide range of biological family members (parents, siblings, grandparents, aunts and uncles, and cousins). We report the prevalence of losses among US children in 2019 by taking all those younger than 18 years in 2019, weighting each single year of age group by its corresponding 2019 population size, and calculating the weighted total and percentage. Our modeling strategy capitalized on new advances in established demographic techniques, including the ability to model experiences of family death from specific causes, using time-varying demographic rates, and separately estimating losing male and female relatives, each of which is important to consider given the dramatic increases in and the gendered patterning of overdose death rates.[4]

Details on these methods, their limitations, and additional analyses are available in the online Appendix. To examine the life course timing of these losses, cohort changes in prevalence, and their gendered nature, we generated age-specific estimates for children younger than 10 years and aged 10 to 17 years, examined these patterns by birth cohort, and separately modeled the deaths of male and female relatives.

RESULTS

We estimated that more than 1.4 million children in the United States experienced at least 1 familial overdose death since birth (Table 1; Appendix Figure A). In total, our results suggest that 1.8% of children in 2019 had experienced such a death. Most strikingly, this percentage

TABLE 1— Estimates of Counts and Percentages of Children Aged Younger Than 18 Years in 2019 Who Had Lost Various Relatives to Overdose Deaths During Their Lifetimes, Overall and by Age Group: United States

	Estimated No. of Children, Thousands (% of Population in Age Group)
Total US population aged < 18 y	77 295.0
Total who experienced kin loss to overdose death	1 421.8 (1.8)
Total who lost ≥ 1 of following to overdose death[a]	
Parents	317.2 (0.4)
Siblings	14.7 (< 0.1)
Grandparents	476.8 (0.6)
Aunts and uncles	536.0 (0.7)
Cousins	89.2 (0.1)
Total US population aged birth to 9 y	39 772.6
Total who experienced kin loss to overdose death	408.0 (1.0)
Total who lost ≥ 1 of following to overdose death[a]	
Parents	85.3 (0.2)
Siblings	1.3 (< 0.1)
Grandparents	164.6 (0.4)
Aunts and uncles	146.2 (0.4)
Cousins	12.6 (< 0.1)
Total US population aged 10–17 y	37 522.4
Total who experienced kin loss to overdose death	1 013.9 (2.7)
Total who lost ≥ 1 of following to overdose death[a]	
Parents	231.9 (0.6)
Siblings	13.4 (< 0.1)
Grandparents	312.2 (0.8)
Aunts and uncles	389.8 (1.0)
Cousins	76.6 (0.2)

Note. All relatives are biological only. Total US population in age group estimates is based on 2019 US Census population estimates.
[a]Not mutually exclusive; could lose more than 1 relative of more than 1 type.

reflects approximately 408 000 children aged younger than 10 years and 1.01 million children aged 10 to 17 years. Although older children experienced overdose losses more frequently, these experiences were patterned by birth cohort, with younger cohorts experiencing much higher rates of overdose loss by each age than older cohorts did, a fact not seen for losses from other causes (Appendix Figures B and C).

The results in Table 1 further demonstrate the wide range of family that children lose to overdose. An estimated 536 000 children (0.7% of the population younger than 18 years) experienced the overdose death of an aunt or uncle, 477 000 (0.6%) experienced the overdose death of a grandparent, and 317 000 (0.4%) experienced the overdose death of a parent, followed by fewer overdose deaths of cousins (0.1%) and siblings (< 0.1%). These patterns were similar across age groups.

Taking a gendered perspective, our estimates confirm that the deaths of male relatives drive the staggering toll of children's overdose loss (Appendix Table A), in line with higher male overdose mortality.[4] Among all children, 926 000 (1.2%) lost a biological father, brother, grandfather, uncle, or male cousin, compared with 503 000 (0.7%) who lost a comparable female relative. Similar male-to-female loss ratios of 2 to 2.5 are seen across both age groups (< 10 years and 10–17 years) and for each focal type of relatives, except grandparents, for whom the ratio is closer to 1.75.

DISCUSSION

Existing data sources are ill-equipped to capture the rates, structure, and experiences of overdose loss among children, leaving this population overlooked in assessments of the overdose crisis. Using recent modeling advances, we reveal the high burden that overdose deaths place on children in the United States, estimating that a staggering 1.4 million children in 2019 had experienced at least 1 family overdose death during their lifetime. Notably, these estimates pertain only to some of the most intimately related family ties—those among children's biological grandparents, parents, aunts and uncles, siblings, and cousins. More children are presumably affected by overdose deaths among other important figures, including unexamined relatives, friends, neighbors, and others. This share would expand further if deaths before a child's birth were considered. The rising burden of loss among children younger than 10 years is especially alarming, portending further growth in this secondary public health threat. Substantial increases in overdose death rates since 2020 further highlight the conservative nature of our estimates. Future work should examine racial, ethnic, geographic, and other disparities in these losses. Scholars also must prioritize the development of culturally sensitive interventions for children's bereavement.

As Athey et al.[1] emphasize, greater attention is needed for the millions intimately affected by overdose deaths—and this brief report serves to remind that this population includes children. Although comparatively few children die of overdose, they are far from passed over by this crisis. The high burden of overdose loss experienced among children is only likely to grow more prevalent as a public health concern. The full consequences of the overdose crisis will continue to define public health for decades to come as these children age into adulthood. AJPH

ABOUT THE AUTHORS

Ashton M. Verdery is with the Department of Sociology and Criminology and the Institute for Computational and Data Sciences, and Cayley Ryan-Claytor is with the Department of Sociology and Criminology, Pennsylvania State University, University Park. At the time of the study, Nilakshi Sarkar was with the Department of Psychology, Pennsylvania State University, University Park. Emily Smith-Greenaway is with the Department of Sociology and the Spatial Sciences Institute, University of Southern California, Los Angeles. Michelle Livings is with the Center for Research on Child and Family Wellbeing, Princeton University, Princeton, NJ.

CORRESPONDENCE

Correspondence should be sent to Ashton M. Verdery, Oswald Tower, The Pennsylvania State University, University Park, PA 16802 (e-mail: amv5430@psu.edu). Reprints can be ordered at https://www.ajph.org by clicking the "Reprints" link.

PUBLICATION INFORMATION

Full Citation: Verdery AM, Ryan-Claytor C, Smith-Greenaway E, Sarkar N, Livings M. More than 1.4 million US children have lost a family member to drug overdose. *Am J Public Health*. 2024;114(12):1394–1397.

Acceptance Date: August 11, 2024.

DOI: https://doi.org/10.2105/AJPH.2024.307847

ORCID iDs:

Ashton M. Verdery https://orcid.org/0000-0003-1005-7580

Cayley Ryan-Claytor https://orcid.org/0009-0002-5728-4975

Emily Smith-Greenaway https://orcid.org/0000-0001-8517-8155

Nilakshi Sarkar https://orcid.org/0009-0004-4444-1382

Michelle Livings https://orcid.org/0000-0002-5916-841X

CONTRIBUTORS

A. M. Verdery designed the study, conducted the data analysis, and wrote the manuscript. C. Ryan-Claytor assisted with designing the study, writing the manuscript, and interpreting the results. N. Sarkar assisted with preparing the data, interpreting the results, and writing the manuscript. E. Smith-Greenaway and M. Livings assisted with writing the manuscript and interpreting results.

ACKNOWLEDGMENTS

We acknowledge support from the National Institute on Aging (1R01AG060949) and the Pennsylvania State University Population Research Institute, which is supported by an infrastructure grant and administers a training program grant from the Eunice Kennedy Shriver National Institute of Child Health and Human Development (P2C-HD041025; T32-HD007514).

Portions of the manuscript were presented at the 2024 Social Networks and Health Workshop of the Duke Network Analysis Center, Duke University, Durham, NC, and the Süßmilch Symposium Lecture of the Max Planck Institute for Demographic Research, Rostock, Germany.

Note. The contents are solely the responsibility of the authors and do not necessarily represent the official views of the National Institutes of Health or other funding sources.

CONFLICTS OF INTEREST

The authors report no conflicts of interest.

HUMAN PARTICIPANT PROTECTION

This study does not use human participant data and is exempt from institutional review board review.

REFERENCES

1. Athey A, Kilmer B, Cerel J. An overlooked emergency: more than one in eight US adults have had their lives disrupted by drug overdose deaths. *Am J Public Health.* 2024;114(3):276–279. https://doi.org/10.2105/AJPH.2023.307550
2. Associated Press, NORC Center for Public Affairs Research. Americans recognize the growing problem of opioid addiction. 2018. Available at: https://apnorc.org/wp-content/uploads/2020/02/APNORC_Opioids_Report_2018.pdf. Accessed March 14, 2024.
3. Sparks G, Montero A, Kirzinger A, Valdes I, Hamel L. KFF tracking poll July 2023: substance use crisis and accessing treatment. KFF. August 15, 2023. Available at: https://www.kff.org/other/poll-finding/kff-tracking-poll-july-2023-substance-use-crisis-and-accessing-treatment. Accessed March 14, 2024.
4. Jalal H, Buchanich JM, Sinclair DR, Roberts MS, Burke DS. Age and generational patterns of overdose death risk from opioids and other drugs. *Nat Med.* 2020;26(5):699–704. https://doi.org/10.1038/s41591-020-0855-y
5. National Institutes of Health. Overdose deaths increased in pregnant and postpartum women from early 2018 to late 2021. November 22, 2023. Available at: https://www.nih.gov/news-events/news-releases/overdose-deaths-increased-pregnant-postpartum-women-early-2018-late-2021. Accessed June 27, 2024.
6. Mason M, Soliman R, Kim HS, Post LA. Disparities by sex and race and ethnicity in death rates due to opioid overdose among adults 55 years or older, 1999 to 2019. *JAMA Netw Open.* 2022;5(1):e2142982. https://doi.org/10.1001/jamanetworkopen.2021.42982
7. Chapman A, Verdery AM, Monnat SM. Opioid misuse and family structure: changes and continuities in the role of marriage and children over two decades. *Drug Alcohol Depend.* 2021;222:108668. https://doi.org/10.1016/j.drugalcdep.2021.108668
8. Jones CM, Zhang K, Han B, et al. Estimated number of children who lost a parent to drug overdose in the US from 2011 to 2021. *JAMA Psychiatry.* 2024;81(8):789–796. https://doi.org/10.1001/jamapsychiatry.2024.0810
9. Schlüter BS, Alburez-Gutierrez D, Bibbins-Domingo K, Alexander MJ, Kiang MV. Youth experiencing parental death due to drug poisoning and firearm violence in the US, 1999–2020. *JAMA.* 2024;331(20):1741–1747. https://doi.org/10.1001/jama.2024.8391
10. Stroebe M, Schut H, Stroebe W. Health outcomes of bereavement. *Lancet.* 2007;370(9603):1960–1973. https://doi.org/10.1016/S0140-6736(07)61816-9
11. Kaplow JB, Saunders J, Angold A, Costello EJ. Psychiatric symptoms in bereaved versus nonbereaved youth and young adults: a longitudinal epidemiological study. *J Am Acad Child Adolesc Psychiatry.* 2010;49(11):1145–1154. https://doi.org/10.1097/00004583-201011000-00008
12. Hamdan S, Melhem NM, Porta G, Song MS, Brent DA. Alcohol and substance abuse in parentally bereaved youth. *J Clin Psychiatry.* 2013;74(8):828–833. https://doi.org/10.4088/JCP.13m08391
13. Fletcher J, Vidal-Fernandez M, Wolfe B. Dynamic and heterogeneous effects of sibling death on children's outcomes. *Proc Natl Acad Sci USA.* 2018;115(1):115–120. https://doi.org/10.1073/pnas.1709092115
14. Patterson SE, Verdery AM, Daw J. Linked lives and childhood experience of family death on educational attainment. *Socius.* 2020;6:1–17. https://doi.org/10.1177/2378023120975594
15. Hulsey EG, Li Y, Hacker K, Williams K, Collins K, Dalton E. Potential emerging risks among children following parental opioid-related overdose death. *JAMA Pediatr.* 2020;174(5):503–504. https://doi.org/10.1001/jamapediatrics.2020.0613

Food Industry Compliance With the Display of Front-of-Package Warning Labels at the Final Phase (2020) of Chile's Labeling and Advertising Law

Natalia Rebolledo, PhD, MSc, Pedro Ferrer-Rosende, MSc, Marcela Reyes, MD, PhD, MSc, Lindsey Smith Taillie, PhD, MPH, and Camila Corvalán, MD, PhD, MPH

Objectives. To investigate food industry compliance with the display of front-of-package warning labels (FOPLs) on products that exceed regulatory thresholds for being high in calories, added sugars, sodium, or saturated fats after full implementation of Chile's Food Labeling and Advertising Law.

Methods. In 2020, trained dietitians took pictures of nutritional information and FOPLs on packaged products in supermarkets. We categorized foods and beverages as requiring FOPLs (or not) using their nutritional composition and ingredients as set out in government guidelines. We compared these classifications with the actual display of FOPLs.

Results. About 62.5% of packaged foods and beverages displayed any FOPL. The most frequent label was for energy (38.7%), followed by sugars (35.2%), saturated fats (26.2%), and sodium (22.6%). Compliance with FOPL display was high (93.6% for any "high-in" designation). Lower compliance was observed in nonsausage meat products (83.5%) and soups (84.5%). Candies and sweet confectionery and sausages contributed most to noncompliance with any "high-in" designation.

Conclusions. Following the law's full implementation, the food industry complied with the display of FOPLs. Mandatory policies with clear guidelines and monitoring systems can contribute to ensuring and sustaining high compliance. (*Am J Public Health*. 2024;114(12):1398–1405. https://doi.org/10.2105/AJPH.2024.307843)

AJPH December 2024, Vol. 114, No. 12

Front-of-package nutrition labels (FOPLs) are defined as labels on the front of food packages providing simple, often graphic, information about nutrients or overall food nutritional quality.[1] FOPLs can guide consumer choices[2] and highlight positive or negative food aspects. When positive, they emphasize product advantages compared with competitors.[3] FOPL regulations are one of the World Health Organization's (WHO's) "best buys" for combating noncommunicable diseases.[4] In addition, the Codex Committee on Food Labeling, a joint initiative of the Food and Agriculture Organization and WHO based in Rome, Italy, establishes standards and guidelines for developing FOPLs for prepackaged foods.[5] However, Codex does not mandate specific labels; thus, several countries have developed their own FOPL systems with various degrees of success.[6,7] A key aspect for evaluating the impact of these policies is to assess industry compliance[8]; however, this is rarely reported.

In 2016, the Chilean government implemented the Food Labeling and Advertising Law, the first regulation to implement FOPLs highlighting negative food characteristics.[9] The law requires that packaged foods and beverages with added saturated fats, sugars, or sodium and exceeding set limits carry a mandatory warning FOPL with the words "high-in" saturated fats, sugars, sodium, or calories. The Chilean Ministry of Health (MOH) created implementation guidelines,[10] while the Health Ministry Regional Secretariat (SEREMI) was responsible for monitoring the law implementation at the food outlet level.

Given that the regulation requires companies to highlight negative food aspects, there was concern about whether the industry would comply with the FOPL use. Thus, in this study, we aimed to investigate the food industry's compliance with the requirement to display FOPLs on packaged products that meet regulatory thresholds for being "high-in" after the law's full implementation in 2020. We examined the proportion of foods high in calories, sugars, sodium, or saturated fats that display the specific FOPLs, reflecting industry compliance with the regulation. This information is also relevant for other countries implementing similar types of FOPL regulations.

METHODS

Chile's law was implemented in 3 phases (June 2016, 2018, and 2019), with progressively restrictive nutrient limits for solids and liquids (Appendix Table A, available as a supplement to the online version of this article at https://www.ajph.org). The law regulates packaged foods and beverages with added saturated fats, sugars, or sodium during processing.[11] Packaged products with added saturated fats, added sugars, or added sodium and exceeding the specified limits for these nutrients or calories must display a FOPL with the words "high-in" and the relevant nutrient. The FOPLs are black-and-white stop signs, and each product can carry up to 4 FOPLs (Appendix Figure A).

The MOH released detailed guidelines for food producers specifying how food products should be labeled, including size, position, and number of labels.[10,12] These guidelines also specified some exceptions. For example, packaged products with a main packaging area greater than 30 square centimeters were required to carry the FOPL directly on the package. However, small products with a main face area smaller than 30 square centimeters were exempt from FOPL in the product itself; instead, the FOPL was placed in the largest container that held them.[12] Another exception involved packaged foods and beverages produced by small and very small food industries. These companies were given a 3-year delay for implementing the law and displayed FOPLs using the first-phase thresholds in June 2019. By contrast, microenterprises are exempted until June 2026.

Chile's Nutrition Facts Panel Database

The Nutrition Facts Panel database contains nutrition information for 13 923 brand-specific packaged products (e.g., chocolate brand 1, chocolate brand 2), photographed from January 14, 2020, to February 27, 2020, after implementing the final phase of the law. Six trained dietitians took photos at 6 to 8 major supermarkets (1 from each of the 6 major national supermarket chains) through an agreement with the Chilean National Association of Supermarkets.[13] We also included 3 candy retailers to increase the variety of candies and sweet confectionery. Using INTAPIC, a software platform with a mobile app developed by our research team, the dietitians scanned product barcodes and took 4 mandatory photos of each packaged food and beverage available in the store: the front of the package, the nutrition facts panel, the list of ingredients, and the warning labels (or a note indicating "no warning label"). After the fieldwork, dietitians reviewed the photos and coded the general identifying information for each packaged product in INTAPIC, following standardized procedures. The information coded included barcode, brand, flavor or other important identifier details, manufacturer, presence of FOPLs, ingredients list, reconstitution instructions, and amount of energy and nutrients (i.e., protein, carbohydrates, total sugars, total fats, fat subtypes if available, and sodium), both per serving size and per 100 grams or 100 milliliters. A supervisor conducted quality control checks and reviewed photographs for accuracy in the data entry.

Data Processing and Definition of the Sample

For products requiring reconstitution (e.g., powdered milk, soups, concentrate juices), we followed package instructions to estimate the energy and nutrient content in the product as consumed. For saturated fats, missing values were replaced by 0 when the total fats content was below 3 grams per portion size, according to local labeling norms. We excluded duplicated packaged products (i.e., duplicates in barcode, name, brand, package size, nutrient composition, and ingredients; n = 2) and products lacking relevant information (i.e., did not include the ingredients list, any information on the amount of energy and regulated nutrients, or reconstitution instructions when needed; n = 122). In addition, we excluded products not under the scope of the regulation (i.e., unprocessed foods, minimally processed foods, culinary ingredients with no increase in the natural content of nutrients of concern as part of their processing, infant formulas, and baby foods without added sugars; n = 3626). The analytic sample included 10 173 products (Appendix Figure B).

Compliance Definition

We defined compliance with Chile's law by verifying the presence of FOPLs on packaged products. Specifically, we first verified whether products were "high-in" based on the MOH guidelines and then compared whether the products displayed the corresponding FOPLs, using the data in INTAPIC. We also categorized products based on the number of "high-in" labels computed from nutrient content data and the number of FOPLs displayed on the packaging. Products were classified into mutually exclusive categories corresponding to 1, 2, 3, or 4 "high-in" designations or 1, 2, 3, or 4 FOPLs. In addition, we categorized packaged products that had at least 1 "high-in" designation or at least 1 FOPL as "any high-in" or "any FOPL," irrespective of the number of labels. It is important to note that our assessment did not extend to other aspects of regulatory compliance such as label placement, size, or additional regulatory criteria.

Verification of the "High-in" Status

We used the verification process described in the MOH guidelines to categorize foods according to Chile's law requirements (Appendix Figure C).[12] The guidelines specify a list of ingredients adding regulated nutrients, including culinary ingredients and food additives that contain sugars, saturated fats, or sodium. We considered food additives as added regulated nutrients regardless of the amount used, even though the guidelines state they should be considered only when added in quantities equal to or greater than 1% of the final product.[12] We determined whether packaged products contained added sugars, saturated fats, or sodium by analyzing the ingredient lists using the R "stringr" package.[14] If a packaged product contained added saturated fats, added sugars, or added sodium and exceeded the specified limits for these nutrients, it was classified as "high-in" the respective added nutrient (i.e., high in saturated fats, high in sugars, and high in sodium). In addition, if a packaged product contained added saturated fats or sugars and exceeded the specified limits for calories, it was classified as "high-in" energy. The full implementation cutoffs for solids or liquids (last column of Appendix Table A) were used depending on the unit of measure displayed on the package by producers (g for solids or mL for liquids).

Food and Beverage Groups

We classified each food and beverage into 1 of 16 mutually exclusive food groups based on previous classifications.[15] The food and beverage groups were beverages (sugar-sweetened, non–sugar-sweetened, and unsweetened); milks and milk-based drinks; yogurts; breakfast cereals (ready-to-eat and to-be-prepared); sweet baked products; desserts, ice creams, and processed fruits; candies and sweet confectionery; sweet spreads; savory baked products; nuts and sweet and savory snacks; savory spreads, seasonings, and dressings; cheeses; ready-to-eat meals; sausages; nonsausage meat products; and soups (powder and ready-to-eat).

Statistical Analyses

We conducted statistical analyses by using R software version 4.1.3 (RCoreTeam, Vienna, Austria). We estimated the prevalence of FOPL by nutrient and number of labels, for the entire sample and each food group. We also estimated compliance (i.e., the proportion of products with FOPLs out of the total number of "high-in" products based on MOH guidelines) by nutrients and for the number of labels, for the entire sample and each food group. Finally, we determined the food and beverage groups with the largest relative contribution to noncompliance within each regulated nutrient category.

RESULTS

After full implementation of the law, 62.5% of the packaged products displayed a FOPL on the packaging. Energy was the most frequent FOPL (38.7%), followed by sugars (35.2%), saturated fats (26.2%), and sodium (22.6%; Appendix Table B). The prevalences of 1 FOPL (22.8%), 2 FOPLs (19.8%), and 3 FOPLs (19.4%) were very similar. Notably, only 0.5% of the products displayed all 4 FOPLs. The proportion of products with FOPLs varied by food group. In some groups, such as sweet baked products, nuts and sweet and savory snacks, and sausages, most products had at least 1 FOPL (97.1%, 92.6%, and 88.4%, respectively). By contrast, in milks and milk-based drinks and yogurts, it was rare to find labeled products (7.1% and 7.7%, respectively).

Food Industry Compliance by Nutrients

In Table 1, we present the compliance by regulated nutrients, overall and by food and beverage groups. Overall, 93.6% of the packaged products were compliant with any "high-in" designation. Among the regulated nutrients,

AJPH December 2024, Vol. 114, No. 12

TABLE 1— Prevalence of Compliance With the Use of Front-of-Package Warning Labels by Regulated Nutrient After the Final Implementation of Chile's Law on Food Labeling and Advertising, Overall and by Food and Beverage Groups: 2020

	Products Identified as "High-in," No.					Compliance, No. (%)				
Food Group	Any "High-in"	Energy	Sugars	Saturated Fats	Sodium	Any "High-in"	Energy	Sugars	Saturated Fats	Sodium
Overall	6589	4146	3584	2688	2352	6168 (93.6)	3835 (92.5)	3426 (95.6)	2501 (93.0)	2181 (92.7)
Beverages	242	1	237	0	5	229 (94.6)	1 (100.0)	224 (94.5)	. . .	5 (100.0)
Milks and milk-based drinks	19	8	16	3	2	17 (89.5)	7 (87.5)	14 (87.5)	2 (66.7)	1 (50.0)
Yogurts	21	3	17	2	4	18 (85.7)	2 (66.7)	15 (88.2)	1 (50.0)	3 (75.0)
Breakfast cereals	274	267	174	62	29	245 (89.4)	240 (89.9)	172 (98.9)	58 (93.5)	27 (93.1)
Sweet baked products	1038	950	914	676	44	1023 (98.6)	932 (98.1)	903 (98.8)	658 (97.3)	38 (86.4)
Desserts, ice creams, and processed fruits	454	222	431	219	6	427 (94.1)	195 (87.8)	412 (95.6)	212 (96.8)	6 (100.0)
Candies and sweet confectionery	1317	1290	1141	680	36	1214 (92.2)	1190 (92.2)	1077 (94.4)	653 (96.0)	32 (88.9)
Sweet spreads	436	193	324	148	93	404 (92.7)	171 (88.6)	313 (96.6)	131 (88.5)	83 (89.2)
Savory baked products	403	343	123	129	161	388 (96.3)	330 (96.2)	119 (96.7)	127 (98.4)	149 (92.5)
Nuts and sweet and savory snacks	367	259	37	59	234	361 (98.4)	255 (98.5)	35 (94.6)	56 (94.9)	229 (97.9)
Savory spreads, seasonings, and dressings	586	226	149	151	470	545 (93.0)	205 (90.7)	126 (84.6)	142 (94.0)	447 (95.1)
Cheeses	349	63	1	95	321	330 (94.6)	55 (87.3)	1 (100.0)	93 (97.9)	304 (94.7)
Ready-to-eat meals	378	115	14	182	288	340 (89.9)	87 (75.7)	13 (92.9)	173 (95.1)	261 (90.6)
Sausages	375	168	0	229	367	350 (93.3)	136 (81.0)	. . .	165 (72.1)	343 (93.5)
Nonsausage meat products	188	19	1	50	154	157 (83.5)	16 (84.2)	0 (0.0)	30 (60.0)	137 (89.0)
Soups	142	19	5	3	138	120 (84.5)	13 (68.4)	2 (40.0)	0 (0.0)	116 (84.1)

Note. Products were categorized as "high-in" using the Ministry of Health Guidelines. Cutoffs correspond to the limits on the amount of energy or nutrient of concern for the full implementation of the law (i.e., for solids, per 100 g: 275 kcal of energy, 10 g of sugars, 4 g of saturated fats, 400 mg of sodium; for liquids, per 100 mL: 70 kcal of energy, 5 g of sugars, 3 g of saturated fats, 100 mg of sodium).

"high-in" sugars had the highest compliance (95.6%), followed by saturated fats (93.0%), sodium (92.7%), and energy (92.5%).

At the food-group level, the highest compliance with any "high-in" designation was observed in sweet baked products (98.6%), nuts and sweet and savory snacks (98.4%), and savory baked products (96.3%). Conversely, the groups with the lowest compliance were nonsausage meat products and soups (83.5% and 84.5%, respectively). The primary compliance issue was "high-in" saturated fats for soups and "high-in" sugars for nonsausage meat products. However, it is important to note that these figures represent small absolute numbers.

Compliance by Number of "High-in" Designations

When analyzing compliance by number of "high-in" designations, we found a limited number of products with 4 "high-in" labels (n = 44). Therefore, these products were grouped with products displaying 3 "high-in" labels (Appendix Table C). Results separated into the 4 categories are available in Appendix Table D.

Overall, compliance was similar and consistent irrespective of the number of FOPLs (3 or 4: 92.7%; 2: 91.2%; and 1: 89.5%). Sweet baked products and beverages consistently achieved high compliance (~95%) regardless of the number of "high-in" designations. Similarly, nuts and sweet and savory snacks had compliance exceeding 95% for 1 and 2 "high-in" designations and more than 90% for 3 or 4 "high-in" designations. By contrast, nonsausage meat products and soups showed lower compliance, approximately 85% or less for any number of "high-in" designations. Sausages and milks and milk-based drinks showed even lower compliance, below 75% for 2 or more "high-in" designations.

Food Groups' Contribution to Noncompliance

When assessing the relevance of each food and beverage group to noncompliance of each label type, we observed that candies and sweet confectionery, sausages, and savory spreads were the primary contributors to noncompliance to any FOPL (Appendix Table E). Specifically, candies and sweet confectionery, sausages, and ready-to-eat meals were the main noncompliers for "high-in" energy. For "high-in" sugars, the leading noncompliant groups were candies and sweet confectionery, savory spreads, and desserts and ice creams. For saturated fats, sausages, candies and sweet confectionery, and nonsausage meat products were most often noncompliant. Lastly, for sodium, the main noncompliant groups included ready-to-eat meals, sausages, and savory spreads.

DISCUSSION

To our knowledge, this is the first study that reports the food industry's compliance with the mandatory display of FOPLs that highlight negative aspects of foods. The Chilean Law on Food Labeling and Advertising mandates the use of FOPLs for products with high content of added sugars, saturated fats, sodium, or calories. Previous studies have shown that consumers are aware that products with more FOPLs are less healthy than those with fewer FOPLs and that consumers use FOPLs when purchasing new products.[16] In addition, the nutritional quality of household purchases has improved.[17] Our study adds to these findings by showing high compliance from the food industry in displaying FOPLs. After full implementation of the law, 62.5% of the packaged products had any FOPL. Overall compliance with FOPL display was high, with 93.6% of products complying with any "high-in" designation, and the lowest compliance was 92.5% for "high-in" energy. Higher compliance was observed in sweet baked products, nuts and sweet and savory snacks, cheeses, and beverages.

Our results suggest that the food industry can modify the packaging to comply with mandatory labeling, even when the law requires displaying unfavorable information. Previous studies from voluntary FOPL policies have shown that the food industry tends to label products to highlight positive aspects, while products with adverse nutrient profiles are labeled to a lower extent.[18–20] For example, the uptake of the Health Star Rating (HSR) system in Australia varied depending on the score received.[18,19] Only 14% of the products with a low HSR of 1.0 displayed the logo, while 49.7% of the products with a high HSR of 5.0 included the logo.[19] In New Zealand, 84% of the products displaying the HSR logo had a higher score between 3.0 and 5.0 stars, whereas the remaining 16% of products with the HSR label had a lower score between 0.5 and 2.5 stars.[20] By contrast, we found high compliance with the display of negative FOPLs, likely because of the mandatory nature of the policy. While the Codex Alimentarius guidelines on nutrition labeling indicate that FOPL policies can be mandatory or voluntary,[5,8] our work demonstrates that mandatory policies are more equitably implemented across the food supply.

Another factor influencing compliance with food regulations is the presence of systems or entities that monitor compliance and apply sanctions to noncompliers. In Chile, the MOH monitored compliance through regional inspections conducted by the SEREMI. The SEREMI targeted venues in which food products were offered (i.e., retailers) rather than the food industry, which was crucial for ensuring the timely and complete implementation of the law.[11] For retailers that did not comply, the MOH initiated legal actions that could result in different sanctions depending on the severity of noncompliance. Sanctions could range from notifications to comply within a stipulated period to monetary fines and prohibition to sell in educational establishments.[21] Although monetary fines could go up to US $145 000, they typically ranged from US $37 to US $3700. The MOH also released reports with findings from the inspections.[21–23] The first report, released 1 year after the initial implementation of the law in 2017, showed that only 64.4% of products complied with the law.[22] For noncompliant products, the MOH started legal actions, with 53.8% of these actions because of FOPL issues. The issues included products without labels, products with labels in an incorrect location, or products with incompatible labeling (i.e., a product with FOPL and health claims). Subsequent reports showed that compliance increased over time. In 2018, 75.2% of products complied with the law, and 36.4% of noncompliance was because of FOPL issues.[23] The experiences from Chile show the importance of having established monitoring systems to achieve compliance with policies.

The high compliance might also be related to the MOH's important role in developing FOPL guidelines that were readily available for producers. Before and during the law's implementation, the MOH released detailed guidelines for food producers, explaining when and how food products should be labeled, including size and position of the FOPL and the number of labels required.[10,12] These guidelines also outlined the compliance verification process with the FOPLs, mentioning that compliance should be evaluated using the ingredients list and nutrient contents, which are mandatory to declare in packaged products.[12,24] Furthermore, the guidelines highlighted specific food groups requiring more attention, such as beverages, sweet and savory snacks, ready-to-eat meals, and dairy products. Our study found that beverages and sweet and savory snacks had high compliance. However, our results suggest that milk and milk-based drinks should be monitored in detail. In addition, nonsausage meat products, soups, and sausages should be added to the list of foods requiring closer monitoring.

Regarding the differences in compliance by regulated nutrients, we found that the "high-in" sugars label had higher compliance than saturated fats, sodium, and calories. It is unclear why compliance was lower for those FOPLs, but 1 potential explanation could be the difficulty in identifying added saturated fats or sodium using the ingredients list. The MOH guideline mentions that a product is categorized as "high-in" saturated fats or sodium only when a mix of food additives is added in quantities equal to or greater than 1% of the final product (if they are the only added source).[12] Given the complexity of defining added saturated fats and added sodium, we may have underestimated compliance for these nutrients because we relied on the ingredients list without knowing the exact amounts of additives in each product. Regarding the "high-in" energy label, a product must have added saturated fats or sugars in the ingredients and surpass the calorie limit to receive this label. Therefore, we could have underestimated the compliance for energy as well.

After the Chilean law was implemented, several Latin American countries adopted similar FOPL policies.[25] However, it is unclear whether our results are generalizable to these countries. We would expect that countries with strong nutritional policies, including mandatory nutrient declaration and robust monitoring systems, might have similar compliance levels to Chile. Yet, there is limited evidence to support this. In Perú, where nutrient declaration is not mandatory, an analysis of 259 packaged products found that 21% of the products did not comply with the regulations. Of these, 35.7% were high in sugars, contained trans fats, or both, but were missing 1 or more warning labels.[26] In México, a country that mandates nutrient declaration, a civil society group reported 2 specific cases of noncompliance, but it is unclear if these were the only cases found.[27] In Uruguay, a review of products from 11 food groups indicated that 47% of cookies were noncompliant.[28] For other products lacking FOPLs, compliance could not be determined because 29% to 62%, depending on the food category, did not provide mandatory nutritional information.[28] In Argentina, there is no information on compliance with FOPL display because monitoring reports have focused on aspects like placement and size.[29,30] This variability highlights the need for more comprehensive studies to understand compliance with negative FOPLs in different regulatory environments. Further research is needed to assess compliance across various settings.

Limitations

This study has limitations. First, we only verified the presence of FOPLs on packaged products without analyzing other aspects of compliance, such as FOPL placement, size, or incompatible labeling. Future studies could include these criteria to strengthen the evidence regarding compliance. Second, the analytic sample included all packaged products available in supermarkets, potentially incorporating those from small, very small, and micro industries. These industries had delayed implementation, which might have led to an underestimation of compliance, as we used the law's third-phase thresholds to classify them as "high-in" regulated nutrients. Future studies could consider industry size when analyzing compliance. Another limitation is the potential overestimation of products "high-in" saturated fats or sodium when considering food additives as ingredients, which would underestimate compliance. Finally, because of data collection agreements, we were unable to analyze compliance by brand, limiting detailed monitoring information.

Public Health Implications

Our findings demonstrate that mandatory FOPL policies can achieve high compliance across different food groups. This suggests that the food industry can adapt to comply with mandatory labeling requirements, even when such policies require displaying unfavorable information about their products. The role of health authorities, such as the Chilean MOH, was crucial in maintaining high compliance levels by monitoring and enforcing compliance. In addition, having clear FOPL guidelines can support food producers in the correct application of labels and facilitate compliance verification. Our results advocate adopting clear guidelines for mandatory labeling policies in other countries, along with establishing robust enforcement mechanisms. Researchers in countries with similar regulations should use available monitoring systems or develop tailored evaluations of labeling compliance as a foundational step for assessing the impact of these policies. AJPH

ABOUT THE AUTHORS

Natalia Rebolledo, Marcela Reyes, and Camila Corvalán are with the Center of Research in Food Environment and Prevention of Obesity and Non-communicable Diseases, Institute of Nutrition and Food Technology, University of Chile, Santiago, Chile. Pedro Ferrer-Rosende is with the Biostatistics Unit, Faculty of Medicine, Universitat Autònoma de Barcelona, Cerdanyola del Vallès, Spain, and the Center of Research in Food Environment and Prevention of Obesity and Non-communicable Disease, Institute of Nutrition and Food Technology, University of Chile. Lindsey Smith Taillie is with the Carolina Population Center and the Department of Nutrition, Gillings School of Global Public Health, University of North Carolina at Chapel Hill.

CORRESPONDENCE

Correspondence should be sent to Camila Corvalán, MD, PhD, MPH, Institute of Nutrition and Food Technology, University of Chile, El Líbano 5524, Macul, Chile (e-mail: ccorvalan@inta.uchile.cl). Reprints can be ordered at https://www.ajph.org by clicking the "Reprints" link.

PUBLICATION INFORMATION

Full Citation: Rebolledo N, Ferrer-Rosende P, Reyes M, Taillie LS, Corvalán C. Food industry compliance with the display of front-of-package warning labels at the final phase (2020) of Chile's Labeling and Advertising Law. *Am J Public Health*. 2024;114(12):1398–1405.

Acceptance Date: August 12, 2024.

DOI: https://doi.org/10.2105/AJPH.2024.307843

ORCID iDs:

Natalia Rebolledo https://orcid.org/0000-0002-4537-6592

Pedro Ferrer-Rosende https://orcid.org/0000-0002-3791-4696

Marcela Reyes https://orcid.org/0000-0002-4601-7663

Lindsey Smith Taillie https://orcid.org/0000-0002-4555-2525

Camila Corvalán https://orcid.org/0000-0003-3766-7709

CONTRIBUTORS

N. Rebolledo and C. Corvalán conceptualized the study. M. Reyes, L. Smith Taillie, and C. Corvalán acquired funding. P. Ferrer-Rosende analyzed the data. N. Rebolledo drafted the article and contributed to data interpretation. All authors critically reviewed and revised the article.

ACKNOWLEDGMENTS

This research was funded by Bloomberg Philanthropies, International Development Research Centre grant 108180 (INTA-UNC) and 107731 (INFORMAS), National Commission for Scientific and Technological Research Fondecyt Regular 1161436, and National Agency of Research and Development Fondecyt Postdoctorado 3230125.

We thank the Chilean National Association of Supermarkets and all the supermarkets and candy distributors involved for authorizing the data collection. We also thank the research teams at the Center of Research in Food Environment and Prevention of Obesity and Non-communicable Diseases at the Institute of Nutrition and Food Technology, University of Chile, and the Global Food Research Program, University of North Carolina at Chapel Hill. We thank Catalina Cornejo and Michelle Vargas for their assistance with data cleaning and food categorization.

CONFLICTS OF INTEREST

The authors have no conflicts of interest to declare.

HUMAN PARTICIPANT PROTECTION

This study did not include human participants. An institutional review board review was not required.

REFERENCES

1. World Health Organization. Guiding principles and framework manual for front-of-pack labelling for promoting healthy diets. 2019. Available at: https://www.who.int/publications/m/item/guidingprinciples-labelling-promoting-healthydiet. Accessed August 28, 2024.
2. Volkova E, Ni Mhurchu C. The influence of nutrition labeling and point-of-purchase information on food behaviours. *Curr Obes Rep*. 2015;4(1):19–29. https://doi.org/10.1007/s13679-014-0135-6
3. Vyth EL, Steenhuis IHM, Roodenburg AJC, Brug J, Seidell JC. Front-of-pack nutrition label stimulates healthier product development: a quantitative

analysis. *Int J Behav Nutr Phys Act.* 2010;7(1):65. https://doi.org/10.1186/1479-5868-7-65

4. World Health Organization. Tackling NCDs: best buys and other recommended interventions for the prevention and control of noncommunicable disease. April 30, 2024. Available at: https://www.who.int/publications/i/item/9789240091078. Accessed September 5, 2024.
5. Joint Food and Agriculture Organization/World Health Organization Codex Alimentarius Commission Codex Alimentarius: Guidelines on Nutrition Labelling CXG 2-1985. Adopted in 1985. Revised in 1993 and 2011. Amended in 2003, 2006, 2009, 2010, 2012, 2013, 2015, 2016, 2017, 2021. 2021. Available at: https://www.fao.org/fao-who-codexalimentarius/sh-proxy/en/?lnk=1&url=https%253A%252F%252Fworkspace.fao.org%252Fsites%252Fcodex%252FStandards%252FCXG%2B2-1985%252FCXG_002e.pdf. Accessed September 5, 2024.
6. Pettigrew S, Jongenelis MI, Jones A, Hercberg S, Julia C. An 18-country analysis of the effectiveness of five front-of-pack nutrition labels. *Food Qual Prefer.* 2023;104:104691. https://doi.org/10.1016/j.foodqual.2022.104691
7. Roberto CA, Ng SW, Ganderats-Fuentes M, et al. The influence of front-of-package nutrition labeling on consumer behavior and product reformulation. *Annu Rev Nutr.* 2021;41(1):529–550. https://doi.org/10.1146/annurev-nutr-111120-094932
8. Sharma LL, Teret SP, Brownell KD. The food industry and self-regulation: standards to promote success and to avoid public health failures. *Am J Public Health.* 2010;100(2):240–246. https://doi.org/10.2105/AJPH.2009.160960
9. Ministry of Health of Chile. Law 20.606: On the Nutritional Composition of Foods and Their Advertising [in Spanish]. 2012. Available at: https://www.bcn.cl/leychile/navegar?idNorma=1041570. Accessed September 5, 2024.
10. Ministry of Health of Chile. Guideline for the Monitoring and Supervision of the Nutritional Composition of Foods and their Advertising, According to the Food Health Regulations [in Spanish]. Santiago, Chile: Nutrition and Foods Department; 2017.
11. Corvalán C, Reyes M, Garmendia ML, Uauy R. Structural responses to the obesity and non-communicable diseases epidemic: update on the Chilean law of food labelling and advertising. *Obes Rev.* 2019;20(3):367–374. https://doi.org/10.1111/obr.12802
12. Ministry of Health of Chile. *Manual for Nutritional Labeling of Foods* [in Spanish]. Santiago, Chile: Nutrition and Foods Department; 2022.
13. Kanter R, Reyes M, Corvalán C. Photographic methods for measuring packaged food and beverage products in supermarkets. *Curr Dev Nutr.* 2017;1(10):e001016. https://doi.org/10.3945/cdn.117.001016
14. Kanter R, Reyes M, Vandevijvere S, Swinburn B, Corvalan C. Anticipatory effects of the implementation of the Chilean Law of Food Labeling and Advertising on food and beverage product reformulation. *Obes Rev.* 2019;20(suppl 2):129–140. https://doi.org/10.1111/obr.12870
15. Dunford E, Webster J, Metzler AB, et al. International collaborative project to compare and monitor the nutritional composition of processed foods. *Eur J Prev Cardiol.* 2012;19(6):1326–1332. https://doi.org/10.1177/1741826711425777
16. Correa T, Fierro C, Reyes M, Dillman Carpentier FR, Taillie LS, Corvalan C. Responses to the Chilean law of food labeling and advertising: exploring knowledge, perceptions and behaviors of mothers of young children. *Int J Behav Nutr Phys Act.* 2019;16(1):21. https://doi.org/10.1186/s12966-019-0781-x
17. Taillie LS, Bercholz M, Popkin B, Reyes M, Colchero MA, Corvalán C. Changes in food purchases after the Chilean policies on food labelling, marketing, and sales in schools: a before and after study. *Lancet Planet Health.* 2021;5(8):e526–e533. https://doi.org/10.1016/S2542-5196(21)00172-8
18. Jones A, Shahid M, Neal B. Uptake of Australia's Health Star Rating System. *Nutrients.* 2018;10(8):997. https://doi.org/10.3390/nu10080997
19. Shahid M, Neal B, Jones A. Uptake of Australia's Health Star Rating System 2014–2019. *Nutrients.* 2020;12(6):1791. https://doi.org/10.3390/nu12061791
20. Mhurchu CN, Eyles H, Choi Y-H. Effects of a voluntary front-of-pack nutrition labelling system on packaged food reformulation: the Health Star Rating System in New Zealand. *Nutrients.* 2017;9(8):918. https://doi.org/10.3390/nu9080918
21. Assessment Report on the Implementation of the Law on Nutritional Composition of Foods and Their Advertising—June 2017 [in Spanish]. Santiago, Chile: Ministry of Health of Chile; 2017.
22. Assessment Report on the Implementation of the Law on Nutritional Composition of Foods and Their Advertising—January 2017 [in Span ish]. Santiago, Chile: Ministry of Health of Chile; 2017.
23. Assessment Report on the Implementation of the Law on Nutritional Composition of Foods and their Advertising—February 2018 [in Spanish]. Santiago, Chile: Ministry of Health of Chile; 2018.
24. Food Health Regulations. Decree No. 977/96 [in Spanish]. Santiago, Chile; Ministry of Health of Chile; 2022.
25. Food Agriculture Organization of the United Nations, Pan American Health Organization, United Nations Children's Fund. Front-of-pack nutrition labelling in Latin America and the Caribbean—guidance note. 2023. Available at: https://openknowledge.fao.org/server/api/core/bitstreams/72c6788c-d339-4f98-9a2f-3b06e01b97f6/content. Accessed September 5, 2024.
26. *Compliance With the Regulations for Including Advertising Warnings on Food Product Packaging in Peru. Technical Reports* [in Spanish]. Washington, DC: Pan American Health Organization; 2021.
27. El Poder del Consumidor. Monitoring the use of characters and warning labels on packaging targeted at girls and boys: preliminary results after the enforcement of the new front-of-package warning label [in Spanish]. 2021. Available at: https://elpoderdelconsumidor.org/wp-content/uploads/2021/06/d-2106-etiquetado-monitoreo-cumplimiento-e-incumplimiento-anexo.pdf. Accessed September 5, 2024.
28. Ministry of Public Health of Uruguay. Supervision of front-of-package labeling [in Spanish]. 2022. Available at: https://www.gub.uy/ministerio-salud-publica/comunicacion/noticias/fiscalizacion-del-rotulado-frontal. Accessed June 5, 2024.
29. Fundación InterAmericana del Corazón Argentina. Monitoring compliance with the healthy eating promotion law during the first months of implementation [in Spanish]. April 27, 2023. Available at: https://www.ficargentina.org/wp-content/uploads/2023/04/2304_reporte_fiscalizacionFOP.pdf. Accessed September 5, 2024.
30. Fundación InterAmericana del Corazón Argentina. Monitoring Compliance With the Healthy Eating Promotion Law [in Spanish]. September 2023. Available at: https://www.ficargentina.org/wp-content/uploads/2023/10/2310_fiscalizacion.pdf. Accessed September 5, 2024.